L.X.F.

Personal Computers
and Special Needs

Personal Computers and Special Needs

FRANK G. BOWE

Berkeley • Paris • Düsseldorf

Cover art by Sato Yamamoto
Book design by Lisa Amon

For Russell Baxter: friend, colleague and teacher.

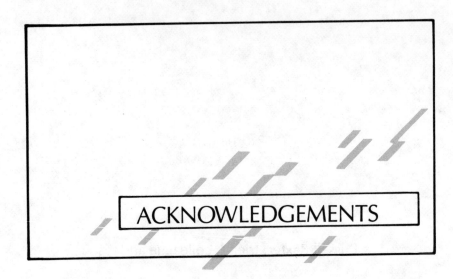

ACKNOWLEDGEMENTS

I acknowledge, with thanks, the work of several friends who helped bring this book into being: Madeleine Will, who took an early interest in the work and assisted in arranging the White House Conference on Computers and Disabled Persons; L. D. Kerr and Lisa D. Williams, who took the pictures in this book; Jim Compton, who read the entire manuscript several times, making numerous helpful suggestions, most of which I adopted; Gregg Vanderheiden, inventor of special-needs keyboard emulators, who read the emulator sections; Jay Rochlin and John Williams, both of whom provided important leads to me. The individuals interviewed for this book gave of their time and knowledge selflessly; their stories contributed a much-needed "high touch" feeling to the book. Most of all, I want to thank "my three girls," my wife Phyllis and daughters Doran and Whitney for putting up with the extensive travel and long hours of writing required to produce this book.

TABLE OF CONTENTS

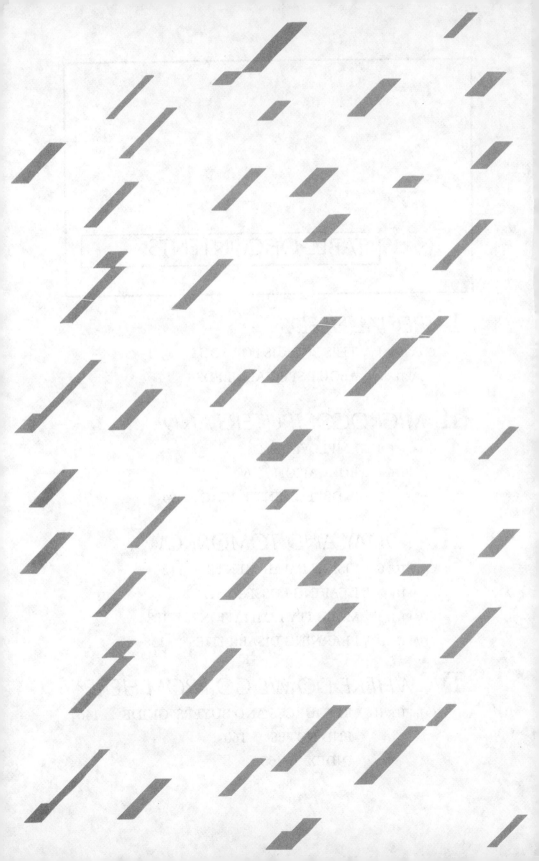

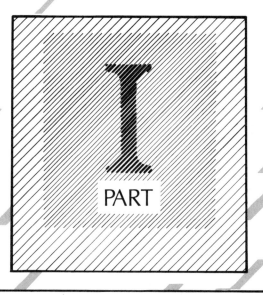

PART I

SPECIAL NEEDS

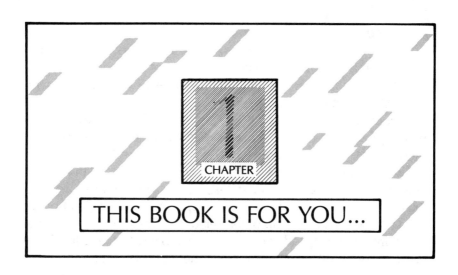

CHAPTER 1

THIS BOOK IS FOR YOU...

I wrote this book for people with special needs, as well as for members of their families and for their friends, co-workers, neighbors, teachers and counselors. If you have a special need, or know someone who does, this book is for you.

Who are people with special needs? The United Nations (UN) estimates that about 10 percent of the world's population is disabled; that is, there are 500 million (one-half billion) persons with special needs. Disabilities, or handicaps, are much more common among people over 65 years of age than among younger people. About one in every eleven under-65 persons is disabled, but the proportion among over-65 individuals is almost one in three. Regardless of when it occurs, disability limits what a person can do. For that reason special needs affect not only the individual but also the family, the class, the office, the organization and the community in which the disabled individual participates. To help attract attention to special needs, the UN has designated the years 1983–1992 as the "Decade of Disabled Persons." National observances are planned in the U.S., the United Kingdom, France, Germany, Japan, and many other nations.

This book is for you . . . if you have a special need. You may not see, hear, move, or learn as well as the others around you. If so, the information in *Personal Computers and Special Needs* will help you to understand how microcomputers can help you overcome your limitations.

This book is for you . . . if you are an adult child beginning to worry about your disabled parents' safety and security. In the U.S., there are more people over 65 (27.4 million) than teenagers (26.5 million), according to the U.S. Bureau of the Census. With medical and nursing-home costs rising so fast, many grown children are anxious to find solutions to their parents' special needs. In this book, I will talk about how to help older persons with special needs live at home much more easily, safely, and enjoyably with the help of personal computers than was possible in the past. Microcomputers can save senior citizens and their grown children considerable amounts of money and time while they reduce worries about accidents, fires and burglaries. Of course, if you are an older person yourself, the same information will help you.

This book is for you . . . if one of your children is handicapped. Education for students with vision, hearing, learning, and mobility restrictions is harder and more demanding emotionally than is schooling for other children. In this book, I will discuss what parents are doing, what kinds of computer programs and games seem to help handicapped children, and how a microcomputer can do things the child cannot do alone. If you are a teacher or a counselor working with handicapped children, the same suggestions may assist you.

And this book is for you . . . if a friend, relative, or co-worker has a special need. You may want to tell him or her about some of the exciting new products now available to meet special needs. If you know something about computers, perhaps you can help this person live and work more easily and effectively.

Finally, this book is for you . . . if you know little or nothing about computers. Until just a few years ago, I was a genuine computer illiterate. I keenly remember how nervous I was when I first sat down at a keyboard. Today, with computers more common and more "user friendly," I figure that most readers of this book are further along the road to computer literacy than I was. But to put to good use the ideas you find here, you don't need to know how a computer's insides work, or how to program a computer. At most, you'll need to call in someone from the store where you bought your machine (such after-purchase support is part of what you get when you buy locally; take advantage of it). Or a friend or neighbor who is more comfortable around electronics can help you. This book will tell you what you need to buy, where to get it, and approximately how much it will cost. This book contains the names and addresses of the organizations and companies that have the specific knowledge and products you will need.

Today, I believe, personal computers are the most remarkable "reasonable accommodation" devices ever invented. Now, there's a term that needs defining. (As we move along, I'll define new terms so you can follow the argument without getting lost.) Several European countries, notably Sweden, the Netherlands, and Germany, have "handicap aids" programs that provide special devices at no charge to eligible individuals. In the U.S., federal laws require schools, hospitals, and employers to provide aids and devices for handicapped students, patients, and workers; the laws call these pieces of equipment "reasonable accommodations" because they provide help at realistic prices. No reasonable accommodation I've encountered, and I've seen almost all of them, is as meaningful to as many people as is the personal computer. A laser cane might help a blind person cross the street, but it does nothing for a deaf individual. A motorized wheelchair helps a quadriplegic office worker to get to and from work, but it offers nothing for someone who is learning-disabled. A microcomputer, on the other hand, helps all of these people.

The concept of reasonable accommodation is one you should remember: if you are a student, client, or employee, some of what's described in this book may be available to you at little or no cost. I will discuss that in considerable detail in the sections of this book that deal with education and employment.

Six years ago, when I first encountered the then-novel notion that microcomputers could help older, handicapped, and chronically ill people, I didn't expect much to happen with these machines. They simply cost too much. Then, you might have to pay $40,000 to $50,000 for a microcomputer-based special-need device. And there were only a few to be had in the entire country. Today, while some aids remain expensive, many devices cost less than $300; some are even priced below $50. Attached to or used with your personal computer, they can do as much as the much more expensive machines once did—or even more.

Six years ago, even three years ago, you were unlikely to hear about these special aids unless you were a regular reader of highly specialized journals or a member of a special-interest group consisting of disabled people. Today you can find many of the aids described in this book in your local hardware store. And, three years ago, you probably had to connect a lot of wires and write complex programs to get the results you wanted. Today often all that's needed is to plug in a device—and away you go.

Despite all of this progress—and it's hard to believe we've come so far so quickly—the majority of people with special needs aren't using personal computers to do the things these machines can be made to do. That's true in the U.S., in Europe, in Japan, and in other regions of the world. Few people with special needs know what microcomputers can do for them. Even fewer know that in some cases they can get what they need at an affordable price or, if they qualify under certain government programs, absolutely free. Others have heard of products they want, but don't know where to get them.

People with special needs must get the information they require in order to free themselves from the shackles of physical, sensory, and learning limitations. That's why I wrote this book: to put in the hands of handicapped people the knowledge that can revolutionize their lives.

And "revolutionize" is not too strong a word to use.

People with limited mobility often need as much as three hours just to get started each morning; reaching light switches, controlling radio dials or television channel switches, and moving about the house or apartment to turn things on and off is time-consuming and difficult for them. A personal computer, with a few add-ons (often called "peripherals," a term that just means devices that are connected to a computer), can save them hours every day. People with chronic health conditions often worry about what might happen in a medical or safety emergency; again, a computer with a few special devices can eliminate much of the worry. Deaf people frequently have to drive miles to reach someone who can help them make a simple phone call; with a computer connected to their phone lines, they can save time and money by making the call themselves.

Microcomputers adapted to meet special needs literally can allow blind people to read. People paralyzed from the neck down can "go to school" and "go to work" without even leaving the home. The difference a personal computer makes can transform a life of passivity, boredom, and fear into one of creativity, productivity, and safety.

The general public often thinks that handicapped people are persons who can't help themselves. That's wrong. With the aid of devices described in this book, even the most severely disabled person can do almost anything he or she did before becoming handicapped.

Equally important, an adapted personal computer can make a person feel much more independent. That means a lot. Instead of having to rely on a grown son or daughter, a nurse, or a personal-care attendant throughout the day, many people can take care of their own needs with minimal assistance from others.

Physically disabled people, especially older people, often spend long hours alone, bored and restless. Computers can provide companionship, entertainment, and personal enrichment. They can help isolated people keep in touch with the world around them.

A dramatic implication of adapted microcomputers is the potential these machines have for helping disabled people to work. If you don't appreciate how much work means to you, try spending six months at home with nothing productive to do. We find challenge, satisfaction, pride of achievement, prestige, and social interaction in work; many disabled people, in fact most such persons, are deprived of all this. In this book, we will "visit" with special-needs persons who use computers to work and learn just how much the new technology means to them.

In fact, the use of adapted personal computers in the employment of disabled people can help countries improve their troubled economies. Particularly in the Scandinavian nations, the United Kingdom, and, to a large extent, the U.S., the costs to support older and disabled persons who do not work are astronomical. Governments often spend more than $10,000 per person per year on aid programs. It would be much less costly to government to provide many disabled persons with adapted microcomputers and to train them for jobs.

As far-reaching as current technologies are proving to be, there are even more exciting developments to come. Within the next five to ten years, personal computers will be able to "hear" conversation—and print out what they hear as they hear it. All of a sudden, telephones, television, radio, and even kitchen-table conversation will become accessible to deaf people. As someone who has not heard a word in three decades, this prospect fills me with a wonderful sense of anticipation. I broke up a congressional hearing last year when I testified that computer speech-recognition would change my life: "Someday soon I'll be able to go to a political rally and hear a politician lie to me."

Also coming is affordable technology that allows a blind person to read virtually anything in print. In fact, such a device exists today: the Kurzweil Reading Machine™. At about $29,000, however, its cost is prohibitive for personal use. Within the next several years, though, the price will drop. You'll place a book, newspaper, or telephone directory on a screen that resembles the glass plate on a copier. A few moments later, you'll hear the text coming out of a speech synthesizer attached to your personal computer. What this will mean for the education and employment of blind and dyslexic individuals is extraordinary.

Today it is often necessary to add components to your microcomputer in order to get done what you need. Within a few years, though, less of that will be necessary. Personal computers will come equipped with built-in speech synthesis and speech recognition capabilities, for example.

What has caused this fast, recent, revolutionary growth in microcomputer technology to help people with special needs? Why, that is, do we now have so remarkably broad a spectrum of personal computer capabilities to meet special needs?

One reason is that personal computers have become amazingly capable, surprisingly inexpensive, and unbelievably popular in a very short time. The capabilities of the microcomputer enable it to do things previously thought to be impossible, and the low cost of personal computers makes these capabilities widely available. And the popularity of the devices makes them the chosen medium for people who want to do something to help handicapped persons.

Let's take an example. Helping people who cannot speak has long been a concern of parents and educators. In years past, they concentrated upon "lapboard and pointer" technologies. The individual used a finger or a wooden pointer to indicate which of an array of printed messages on the board he wanted to communicate (e.g., "drink"). Today, instead of trying to invent a better message board, parents, teachers and interested technicians are working on computer programs and peripherals. A computer with a speech synthesizer, for example, lets a nonvocal individual "speak" more satisfyingly complete sentences much faster and with more ease than is possible with a message board.

Ten years ago, even five years ago, inventors wanting to help deaf people use the telephone worked with the decades-old teleprinter technologies. The resulting devices, called, at first, teletypewriters (TTYs) and later, telecommunications devices for the deaf (TDDs), enabled deaf people to call others who had similar equipment, but no one else. Figure 1.1 shows a TDD. Today microcomputers

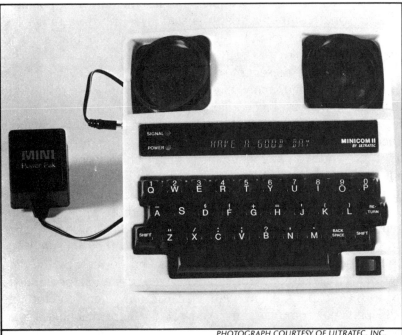

PHOTOGRAPH COURTESY OF ULTRATEC, INC.

Figure 1.1: The Minicom II^{TM}, a popular telecommunications device for the deaf (TDD), costs about $150.

are used so that deaf people who own personal computers can call others who own such machines as well as people still using TDDs.

Three years ago, education for learning-disabled children and youth focused on the demanding process of breaking through the limitation: dyslexic students, for example, were taught how to read. Today, educators realize that the ability of computers to produce spoken versions of words and data frequently makes it possible for such children to hear what they do not understand through vision. When such devices become more widely available, they will make a remarkable difference in the quality of education the children receive. In the past, the teaching of other subjects had to be delayed for several years while educators concentrated on the arduous task of instruction in reading; in the future, academic teaching may be concurrent with instruction in reading.

It is only recently that the personal computer has become a staple in everyday life. But, as quickly as this happened, disabled persons and scientists moved, just as quickly, to tap the emerging potential. The personal computer, they realized, was more versatile, less costly, and more beneficial a technology to work with than anything previously available.

There's another reason for so many special-needs devices. Fifteen or twenty years ago, many parents and educators were resigned to the inevitability of a limited life for a handicapped child or youth. Beginning in the late 1960s, however, parents in particular began to become much more assertive and demanding. They took educators to court—and won victories assuring their children of the right to attend public schools. They went to Washington—and got Congress to pass the Education for All Handicapped Children Act of 1975 (P.L. 94–142). And many parents, particularly those with engineering and mechanical skills, refused to accede to a child's limitations; rather, on their own or with friends and colleagues, they invented first crude, and then more sophisticated aids and devices. By the time the 1980s rolled around, these parents were using microcomputers to do their experimenting with, because they were comfortable with personal computers and knew what these machines could do for their children.

However, much of the progress is due to none of these factors.

Speech recognition, for example, began not because someone wanted to help deaf people understand the spoken word but because business executives, who control the purchase of most business-use computers, do not like to type. They would much rather talk to a secretary, who would then do the typing. Computer companies quickly realized that the key to big sales lay in enabling the executive to dictate to a computer as he or she does to a secretary. As the work began, the implications of speech-recognition technology for deaf people became evident. But it was always, and still is, a secondary consideration. Much the same happened with speech synthesis. Today, your car talks to you ("Close the door") and so do many soda machines. The remarkable omnipresence of talking devices is due not to a desire to help blind people so much as to the need to make machines "user friendly."

The motivations of the inventors and manufacturers are irrelevant to most of us. The important thing is that the machines we need are here or on the way. In fact, it is probably fortunate for people with special needs that their particular requirements converge so neatly with the desires of the general public, because there were some special problems with the "special devices" designed and manufactured only for handicapped people.

Because the market was relatively small, mass production of such devices was impossible. Hence, the price per unit was high. I remember, six years ago, talking with Dr. Howard Rusk, then director of the New York University (NYU) Institute of Rehabilitation Medicine in Manhattan, about an "NYU wheelchair" invented by members of his staff. This electronic wheelchair was truly remarkable. It could "hear" and "understand" about 80 two-word commands. Rusk's staff had designed the chair for people who had been paralyzed by automobile, diving, or sports accidents, but who could talk. The NYU wheelchair would turn on the television, for example, in response to the command: "TV on." As impressive as the device was, and as needed as it surely still is, it could not be mass produced because of the small market for it and its cost, for each chair, of $35,000. At that price, I was not surprised to learn that there were only two such wheelchairs in the country.

Now, let's contrast this situation with what's known as "BSR technology." You can get a BSR home-control console in your local hardware store. It operates, by remote control, more than a dozen devices in the home and costs $40. There are millions of them around today. And the reason for the low cost, widespread availability, and convenience of purchase is that the BSR console was designed for, and is sold to, the general public, not the special-needs population. My point: who cares? The device allows someone with a special need to do more, much more, than he or she could possibly do with a special device just a few years ago—and at a dramatically lower price.

Special devices had another problem—they were difficult to get repaired. Because most were made by small firms, a malfunctioning device had to be returned to the manufacturer for repair. Sometimes these firms went bankrupt before the device you bought needed repair. There was no one else around who knew how to fix the thing. General-use devices that are accessible to people with special needs, however, share few, if any, of these difficulties. Usually, you can get it repaired in your own hometown. In some cases, the cost to repair the aid would exceed the price of a new one, so you'll just buy another.

Today, what once was "special" rapidly is becoming "general." ComputerLand™ stores, for example, now carry touch pads, speech synthesizers and speech-recognition devices, all of which were once "special needs" aids. The computer-store chain has found that many nondisabled individuals feel more comfortable with computers when they can avoid the keyboard and interact directly with the machine. Koala™ pads that let users draw with a stylus or finger on a special surface once were marketed by Koala Technologies Corp. primarily to special-education programs; today, the growing company sells the $150 touch pads to nondisabled children and adults who feel they are more "user friendly" than keyboards. One year ago, speech recognition products primarily were sold to people who could not use keyboards at all, including individuals with severe physical disabilities as well as manufacturing-plant inspectors whose jobs required them to walk rapidly through plant floors. Now, however, products that "hear" are being marketed by such companies as Texas Instruments and Voice Machine Communications to local computer stores for the general market. Some observers predict that within three years, one out of every four computers sold will be equipped with some kind of "special" aid or device. For people with special needs, that is welcome news because it means the products will be more easily repaired, more readily available, and much less expensive than they were just one or two years ago.

I'll introduce you to these aids and devices in this book. You will learn what people in the U.S. and Europe are doing with microcomputers, how they are doing these things, and how you can do them too. I'll tell you where to buy the aids you want. You'll see what you can expect to pay to get the functions you need. And you'll find out where to turn for more information. Usually, I'll give you an address immediately after I discuss a product or service, so you'll have the resources available when you want them.

This is not a book on theory; I'll leave that to the academicians. Rather, my focus is on concrete facts: what you can do and how you can do it.

It is not a book on engineering or computer programming; you don't have to be an electronics engineer or a programmer to benefit from the information in these pages. In some cases, you might want to call in someone in your town who can help you attach the various components, but knowing who to ask is about all you'll have to bring to the ideas you'll find in this book.

And it is not a book endorsing any particular manufacturer's products. It is true that many of the special programs now available were written originally for use with Apple computers. This is primarily because Apples were so popular during the first several years of the so-called personal computer revolution. But you'll see that TRS 80®, Commodore 64™, IBM PC™, Osborne I® and other computers now can do a lot for you. And it is true that some firms, such as Ohio's Prentke Romich, have dominated the peripheral market for special-needs devices in recent years. Since then, however, many other companies have entered the field. I'll tell you what's available and show you how individual people use these devices, but please bear in mind that none of the machines mentioned in this book is endorsed or recommended over others by the author or by the publisher.

Rather, this is a book that responds to the real needs many people have for help with problems that can overwhelm them and their families, by offering objective information they can use to solve practical, everyday problems.

When I start on a long trip, I like to look over a road map to get some idea of what I'll be encountering along the journey. When I read a book, too, I like to know, quickly, what is and is not between the covers.

Chapter 2 talks briefly about different kinds of special needs. Some readers won't have to read this chapter; they already know all they need to know about their own needs. But parents, educators, counselors, friends, and relatives might want to know more about special needs in order to understand how the devices described in this book can meet those needs.

The next section, Part II, takes up specific problems: employment, education, and independent living. Here I'll consider what computers can and cannot do. Interviews with disabled people who use microcomputers will illustrate these capabilities and show how the technologies work in actual practice.

In Part III, I'll review the ways that microcomputers can help people with different kinds of special needs: blindness, deafness, mobility limitations, and learning limitations. I'll share with you information about international and domestic organizations that specialize in assisting persons with these limitations, so you'll know where to turn for help.

The final section of this book, Part IV, offers product and service information. You'll find a discussion of resources, such as users' groups, information and referral organizations, and special-interest publications. Then I've provided a detailed table that summarizes hardware, software, and resources information in handy form. The table brings together much of the information that's offered in narrative form in earlier parts of the book.

Now, a note about myself. I've used many of the computers discussed in this book. Those I haven't personally used, I've seen in operation by people with special needs. For several years now, as a consultant to the U.S. Congress and to various other international and domestic organizations, I've watched the emergence of special-needs capabilities in microcomputers. And while executive director of the so-called "handicapped lobby," the American Coalition of Citizens with Disabilities (ACCD), I came to know thousands of people with special needs. Many became my friends. I've kept in touch with them and have shared their sense of excitement as they began using personal computers to make their lives easier, more productive, and more fun. When I decided to write this book, they helped me understand what microcomputers could do—for you.

Perhaps few things illustrate more vividly how much personal computers are changing the lives of disabled people than the careers of my staff members after I left ACCD. My director of research is now a manager in a major computer corporation. The man who ran my public relations department now heads Technical Communications Inc., where he publishes a monthly paper, *Special Needs Computing,* which monitors access to "The Information Age" much as the ACCD newsletter used to track access to transportation. Another staff member became vice president for planning at a major forestry trade association, where he uses computers for creating "what if?" scenarios. And my sign-language interpreter took an MBA at Columbia University and is now a banking executive who uses spreadsheet programs on her personal computer.

If what I've described sounds interesting, this book is for you.

CHAPTER 2

ABOUT SPECIAL NEEDS

In the United States today, approximately 27 million to 36 million people are disabled. A little more than 4 million are under the age of 16. More than 13 million are aged 16 to 64, and 8 million are over the age of 65. And another 2 million of all ages reside in institutions. These figures reflect only those persons the U.S. Bureau of the Census and other federal agencies have counted or projected. It is reasonable to expect that some people who have disabilities do not report them to census takers; so the true figure may be as high as 36 million.

The rate of disability in a body of people varies greatly depending upon how old these persons are. Only one in every twenty-seven individuals aged 16 to 24, for example, reports a disability; among persons aged 65 to 74, however, nearly three in every ten declare that they have a disability. Most people with disabilities were once able-bodied; most, in fact, worked before an illness or accident disabled them.

If you talk to these people, as I have, you learn quickly that most are healthy. Someone may have been blinded in an accident ten years ago, for example, but aside from that is in excellent health.

And most want to work and to remain active in the community.

Yet the facts are inescapable: the vast majority of people with special needs do not work. Take American working-age (16–64) women who have disabilities, for example: the proportion at work is just one in five. About one-third of disabled men of the same age range work. Fewer than one in ten disabled men and one in fifteen disabled women over 65 years of age work. In Europe, the proportion of persons with disabilities at work is even lower than it is in the U.S.

Most disabled people are not working for several reasons. The major cause is probably employer bias: people with special needs often face discrimination in the workplace. Employment interviewers just do not believe that these persons can and will work as well as do persons without any special needs. The tragedy is that they are so wrong. As DuPont, IBM, AT&T, Control Data, and other corporations have shown in the U.S., with some basic "reasonable accommodation" aids and devices, such as those described in this book, people can handle their special problems well enough to unleash their abilities for productive work. In Great Britain, Remploy Ltd. has demonstrated the same thing, with 9,000 disabled workers at 94 factories throughout the country.

Another reason more do not work is that their personal lives are difficult and demanding. Physical impairments, for example, make doing the simplest chores around the house exhausting; the same restrictions make commuting to and from work problematic. With the kinds of aids described in these pages, many such people can gain enough control over their personal lives to be free to work.

That it can be done is demonstrated by the hundreds of thousands of disabled men and women who work full-time and lead active personal lives as well. They are, by and large, not "superachievers." Rather, they've learned how to use aids and devices to compensate for their limitations—and they've been able to convince employers to hire them. The relatively few who get year-round full-time jobs earn nearly as much as do their able-bodied colleagues. It can be done—and often is. With the devices described in this book, it can be done by many more people.

On an average day, about 1,200,000 people are in American nursing homes. Thousands more enter such homes each year because they can no longer live independently. For many, it is very traumatic. Several times as many older persons move from their home into another home, often to live with their grown children. Again, such a move is difficult for many elderly people to make. Some of the devices described in this book can delay for several years the necessity for such wrenching relocations. We cannot put a dollar value on what it means to many older persons to be able to remain at home, comfortable, safe, and secure.

Let's look at some of the restrictions or limitations that disabled people face.

Vision Impairment

Stephen Rogers is a professor of liberal studies at the University of Notre Dame, where he has taught for 20 years. He earned his Ph.D. in comparative literature at Harvard and has written extensively on modern mythologies, romantic poetry, and Shakespeare. He is also legally blind. Dr. Rogers uses an Apple II Plus® equipped with an Echo II™ speech synthesizer to do his voluminous writing and editing work. The Echo lets him listen to words he can't read: it converts print to sound. In effect, Rogers uses the Echo as a "monitor" (hearing rather than seeing what he's writing) and the Apple as a word processor. "More than once, I've stayed up until 4:00 A.M. with the computer," he says. Rogers' 11-year old daughter uses the speech synthesizer to make computer games more enjoyable, but only when her father isn't at the machine. Rogers says:

> For years, writing has been one of my professional duties; it is a task I sometimes love and sometimes hate. Although I have had lots of good help from readers [sighted persons who read aloud for him] and especially from my wife, I have been frustrated, at times almost intellectually paralyzed, by the numerous gaps between my thoughts and the pages I wrote.

Now all that is changed: "It is the freedom of composition that makes the real difference. Never have I had such control over what I write."

Rogers is one of about 1.7 million blind persons in America. Legal blindness is 20/200 vision after correction; that is, a blind individual can see at 20 feet what a sighted individual can see at ten times that distance. Vision impairment is common among older Americans, as sight is one of the capacities that deteriorate with age. A total of about 11 million people of all ages in the U.S. have impaired vision; most, however, can see fairly well with glasses or other aids. In some cases, surgery can restore usable vision.

A popular misconception is that most blind people read Braille. In fact, only about one in every ten does. The reason is basic: loss of vision usually occurs later in life. Rather than attempt to learn a difficult skill that would be of limited help, most blinded individuals rely on tape recorders and human readers to keep up with paperwork. Today they can use speech synthesizers, such as Rogers' Echo.

A speech synthesizer helps a blind person in a number of ways. One of the most important is in the acquisition of information. Words and data stored on a computer, entered by the blind person or by others, may be retrieved and "read" almost as easily and quickly by a blind person as by a sighted one. Rogers points out, though, that "it is still faster for sighted people to read a screen than it is for me to listen to the synthesizer." Devices like the Echo are particularly helpful for students and workers who must keep up with large quantities of information. But they help enrich the lives of others as well, simply by greatly expanding the person's ability to maintain contact with the community.

A second way synthesizers can help is illustrated by Rogers' use of his Apple: using special software, Echo can read out entire words. For writing and editing, a word processing program especially written to be used with the Echo II can spell out those words and even indicate punctuation. Such capabilities are invaluable.

Blind people encounter prejudice in the labor market. I wish I had five cents for every time a blind person has told me about losing out on a job opportunity because the interviewer said: "You can't keep up with the paperwork." With a microcomputer and a speech synthesizer, blind individuals can, in fact, handle large doses of information quickly and efficiently; they need no longer restrict themselves to stereotyped jobs, such as piano tuners, musicians, and the like.

But what blind individuals tell me over and again about speech synthesizers is how these devices make them feel independent. To appreciate the depth of feeling they bring to those statements, consider the imposition of having to rely upon a human reader to get through your business and personal papers; in addition to the frequent invasion of privacy, there is the not inconsiderable matter of dependency on another person. Rogers, for example, is an enthusiastic proponent of microcomputers equipped with speech synthesizers: "I have an extravagant hunch that every print-handicapped person in school or the professions would benefit from having access to a talking computer."

Hearing Loss

Karen Maliszewski is a slender 13-year-old who likes swimming, mathematics, and art. A student at Lewis and Clark Junior High School in Omaha, Nebraska, Karen struggles to keep up with her 1,100 fellow students, although she has an I.Q. of 140. Karen is deaf. Deafness occurring early in life interferes with the natural and effortless task most children perform, almost without thinking about it: acquiring a mastery of the English language.

Karen found computers helpful when she spent a recent summer as one of 27 deaf campers at Boys Town in Nebraska. The ability of a microcomputer equipped with a spelling-checker program to help her with her writing made the difficult job of learning language easier and more enjoyable for her.

Two million Americans of all ages are deaf. Deafness is the inability to hear and understand conversational speech through the ear alone. Most deaf people rely on lipreading or sign language for interpersonal communication, and upon reading for information acquisition. A total of 400,000 deaf people lost their hearing before they reached employment age. For most of these individuals, learning to read and write well was very difficult. Today's computer "dictionaries" help by automatically identifying the misspelled words in a text, as illustrated in Figure 2.1. Some software just now coming on the market allows them to improve their prose by substituting less familiar synonyms for words they know well but use too often for their writing to read smoothly. We are even beginning to see computer software that corrects grammar and syntax. These products are useful to the general public as well as to people who are deaf: for this reason, most are much more affordable than they would be if designed only for use by deaf individuals. Spelling and grammar programs are of enormous benefit to people like Karen, who often are embarrassed to show others what they've written.

That's not all computers can do for people who are deaf. With a modem (modulator-demodulator; basically, an interface, or go-between, for connecting a computer with a telephone wire), a computer becomes a machine that a deaf individual can use to communicate by phone with others who have computers. And with information services such as The Source™ and CompuServe™, they can hook into electronic mail. Another attachment, which permits the machine to function both as an "eight-level" (ASCII; American Standard Code for Information Interchange) device—that is, like a computer—and as a "five-level" (Baudot) machine—that is, like a traditional TDD—allows deaf people to telephone friends who have TDDs as well as others who use microcomputers.

By the time Karen enters the labor market, personal computers may be able to understand continuous speech. If so, she could use a microcomputer to function fully independently on the job and at home.

Ernie Hairston is a deaf professional who uses a Tandy Radio Shack 4P™ personal computer at work and at home. An educational media specialist with the U.S. Department of Education in Washington, he wrote *Black and Deaf in America* with the late Linwood Smith, another man who was both deaf and black. Figure 2.2 shows Ernie with his portable computer.

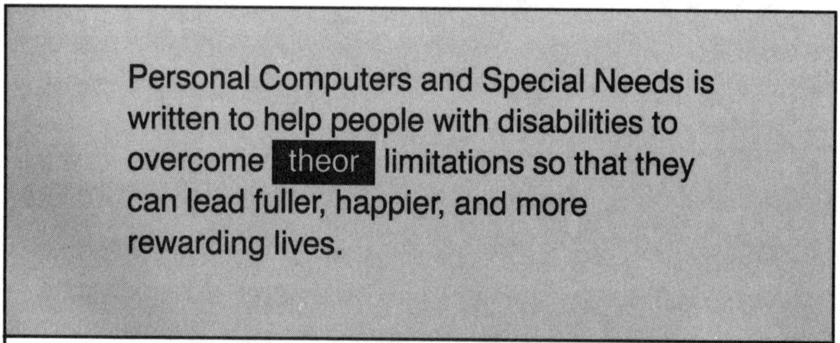

Personal Computers and Special Needs is written to help people with disabilities to overcome theor limitations so that they can lead fuller, happier, and more rewarding lives.

Figure 2.1: *A spelling checker program helps the user locate all the misspelled words in a document.*

Mobility Limitation

John Collins is an entrepreneur in northern Virginia. Owner of Van Go, a privately held corporation, John uses an Osborne I portable computer to maintain the books for his company and perform mailing-list services for his clients. John has myositis ossificans progressiva, a rare calcium disease that immobilizes most of his limbs. From a motorized wheelchair, he uses his Osborne to store, retrieve, and manipulate words and data far faster and much easier than he was able to with conventional typewriters and paper. "My computer has made it possible for me to increase my business and have fun while doing it," he says.

John made some adaptations to the Osborne I he bought two years ago. He uses a four-foot extension cord to permit him to place

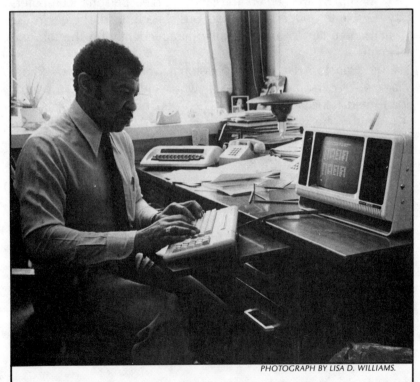

PHOTOGRAPH BY LISA D. WILLIAMS.

Figure 2.2: Ernie Hairston with Tandy Radio Shack 4P™ portable computer in his office.

the keyboard on his wheelchair lapboard. And because he sits too far away from the computer to read its small display, he added a larger, separate monitor that hangs at eye level on the wall next to his computer.

John Collins is one of approximately ten million Americans who have mobility limitations, usually in the upper or lower limbs. Almost all of these people, unlike John, can walk with simple aids and devices, such as canes, crutches and braces. About 500 thousand use wheelchairs.

Safety and health considerations are important to people with mobility restrictions. Microcomputers can help them in a number of ways. With a modem and an automatic telephone dialer (a device that obviates the necessity of dialing; it enables the computer to call up a telephone number from its memory and dial the number itself), emergency medical, fire, or burglar alarm signals may be issued directly to the approprate persons or organizations.

Using The Source, CompuServe, or similar information services, a person with a severe mobility limitation may eliminate many trips out of the home. Coming soon are "videotex" services which will allow shopping from the home; in Florida and a few other states, such services already are commercially available. Some banks, such as Citibank in Manhattan, offer home banking services to customers for a modest monthly fee. (Videotex and home-banking services are not, of course, specifically designed for disabled people; they are attractive time-savers for millions of able-bodied individuals.) Taken together, these microcomputer capabilities can dramatically reduce the number of "errand" trips a person has to make. For disabled people, they will conserve time and strength while alleviating concerns about safety.

And, as John Collins demonstrates, personal computers can help many previously "unemployable" people find and perform well-paying work.

Learning Disability

Kevin Myers, a 14-year-old who lives in Scottsdale, Arizona, experienced difficulty in school because of a learning disability. "He was more capable of retaining auditory stimuli than visual stimuli," says his father, Dr. Gerald Myers. Myers equipped the family Heath H-89™ computer with a Votrax™ speech synthesizer, so Kevin could listen to lessons instead of trying to read them. Then Dr. Myers went further, writing an interactive program he called "Nivek" (for Kevin, spelled backwards) that helps Kevin practice his mathematics skills.

Dyslexic individuals have difficulty comprehending what they see, particularly printed words. Other, less common, learning disabilities interfere with the ability to understand what is heard. Learning-disabled people almost always have normal intelligence, vision, and hearing.

Education for children with learning disabilities is demanding—and expensive. Pine Woods School in Williston, Vermont, for example, offers individual instruction and small classes, stressing alternative ways of using brain cells to acquire functions, such as reading, that are impaired by the disability. Enrollment costs, in 1983, averaged nearly $15,000 a year.

For people like Kevin Myers, the personal computer opens up a whole new world: almost effortless learning. And it provides a way of working effectively and quickly despite a learning disability.

Mental retardation is different from such impairments. Retardation is a general reduction in intellectual functioning. People who are retarded usually respond better to what they hear than to what they read; some do not learn to read at all. Many can acquire an impressive number of skills, but usually only after long hours of repetitive practice.

For persons who are retarded, the computer provides a patient, uncritical tutor; equipped with a speech synthesizer, it can talk to the student. And, with appropriate programming, the computer can be used to remind a retarded person what to do and how to do it, thus enhancing the ability to live independently.

A Dissenting View

Not all people with special needs welcome the advent of personal computers adapted to meeting these needs. This is hardly surprising, given the fact that many Americans and Europeans still fear or even loathe computers.

Irving K. Zola, a professor of sociology at Brandeis University and physically disabled himself, is distrustful of the concept of "doing too much technically." He observes, for example, that his leg brace has a tendency to cause pressure sores. Zola solves the problem by placing a small patch over the spot every day. He notes with a sense of pride that his orthopedist, who would prefer to design a custom brace, views the adaptation dubiously. "I have solved something they could not," he says. "But I have also done something else. I've made the brace more a part of me because I have given it my own unique stamp."

Dr. Zola does not advocate the elimination of mechanical and electronic aids; far from it. But he does inject a needed dose of psychology into the realm of aids for people with special needs. "My point is a simple one, that care, as in the terms 'medical care' or 'personal care', is not merely a technical task," Zola says. "To objectify this care into a technical service, to replace the human element with a mechanical or animal one, can only lead to further objectification of the individual receiving that service."

As I move on to consider the ways in which personal computers can be used to help people with special needs, Dr. Zola's observations should not be forgotten. Whether helping an elderly parent remain at home, a handicapped child learn in school, or a disabled adult perform work, the objective is always to help people help themselves.

There is an old Chinese proverb that illustrates this point nicely: "Give a man a fish, and he will eat for a day. Teach him how to fish, and he will eat for the rest of his life." What Dr. Zola is saying is that *he* needs to do something to retain his sense of self-worth. Were a machine to do everything for him, leaving no room for him to express his individuality and creativity, he would feel devalued. Thus, something as small as placing a patch on a sore spot becomes important because it permits exactly this assertiveness. John Naisbitt makes a similar point in his book, *Megatrends*. Nasibitt argues that high technology almost always fails to win popular approval unless "high touch" features also are offered. When banks tried to convert customers to electronic funds transfer, for example, people resisted the change; they wanted to do something themselves. Naisbitt says he feels virtuous writing out checks but "now the banks want to take that away from me."

The tremendous potential of microcomputers should not obscure from our view the desires of people to maintain their dignity and independence.

The Limits of the Possible

The personal computer field is bedeviled by a rash of compatibility problems. When two things work together, they are said to be "compatible." The Echo II speech synthesizer that Dr. Rogers uses, for example, is compatible with an Apple II Plus computer. Similarly, the software John Collins uses with his Osborne is compatible with that machine. Just as people must use leaded or unleaded gasoline, depending on the make and model car they drive, so too must people who have a computer use software and hardware that work with that computer. The usual advice to people interested in buying their first computer is to first select the software that meets their needs and then pick a computer that runs that software. It is good advice. For most people, a personal computer is actually just a medium for running software. It is the software, the computer program, that really does the work: the word processing, the calculating, the graphic imaging that you want done. If, to illustrate, your needs are best met by the Lotus 1-2-3™ program, you are well advised to shop for a computer that is compatible with this program.

People with special needs who use peripherals face still more compatibility problems. The Echo II speech synthesizer, for example, is not compatible with "protected" software, such as WordStar™ by MicroPro. Dr. Rogers could not use the Word-Star word-processing program designed to run on Apple II Plus computers because the speech synthesizer won't vocalize the text created with the WordStar program. That's why he had to use a software program written specifically for use with the Echo II synthesizer.

The problem is not unique to speech synthesizers. Severely disabled children with cerebral palsy, for example, sometimes use a specially designed message board to enter words and data into a personal computer. Message boards are easier for these children to manipulate than are standard computer keyboards; for example, the individual keys are much larger and more widely spaced. Some boards allow the user to enter entire words or strings of words with just one command. I watched as one child played a computer game with a message board. When she tried to play a second game, however, nothing happened: the new game was not compatible with her message board.

People who need peripherals should consider these compatibility problems carefully. Disabled individuals I've talked to tell me that first they decided what they wanted to do with personal computers. They asked themselves such questions as: Is my major interest word processing or is it calculating? Then they looked for peripherals that would meet their special needs. Some blind people like to listen to information, so speech synthesizers were the aids they investigated; other blind individuals prefer to read Braille, so machines that produce Braille output attracted their interest. Only then did they look at software programs on the market to find those they could use with the peripherals they had selected. The question of which computer to purchase was then answered by asking: What computer is compatible with *both* the peripherals I need and the software programs I want? The special-needs device became the starting point, the core around which they built their system.

These problems may be resolved in the years to come. In February 1984, representatives of AT&T Bell Laboratories, International Business Machines, Apple Computer, Tandy Radio Shack, and Honeywell met at a White House Conference on Computers and Handicapped Persons to discuss how to make hardware and software more accessible to people with disabilities. If these manufacturers can eliminate some of the compatibility problems now frustrating disabled persons, people like Stephen Rogers will have a much broader selection of products from which to choose. That would be a major step forward. Of the more than one hundred word-processing programs on the market today, Rogers can use only one or two. Someday soon, he may be able to use dozens.

A different set of concerns arises from the limited memory of many computers. Personal computers do not have as much memory as do larger, mainframe computers; they can't "remember" as much and they don't have as much "room" to explore. Computer memory comes in two basic kinds: "read-only memory" (ROM) and "random-access memory" (RAM). ROM represents a computer's permanent memory: it contains basic instructions, sets of data, and other information the computer needs to do its work. RAM, on the other hand, is temporary memory. When you do word processing on a computer, for example, the commands you use trigger the computer's ROM, which in turn tells the computer what to do to implement your commands. The words you type, however, go into the RAM.

Suppose, for example, you wanted to use speech recognition with your computer. Perhaps you have a severe physical disability that makes typing extremely difficult. Talking to the computer is much easier for you. There are speech-recognition products on the market today that function very well. But, because of the sharply limited memory of most personal computers, it is only possible to say a few words to the computer. It does not have enough memory to store instructions for translating more than a handful of spoken words. Similarly, most speech-recognition products available today have enough memory only to store the way one person pronounces those words. If another individual speaks to the computer, nothing will happen.

The emergence of more powerful small computers may help resolve memory problems, because such computers have many more times as much memory as do most personal computers. Eventually, small computers will be capable of recognizing continuous speech. Today the new 32-bit computers, such as Apple's Lisa™ and Macintosh™ computers, are more powerful (have more memory) than smaller, 16-bit or 8-bit microcomputers. AT&T's new 3B™ computers, similarly, are 32-bit machines.

As an example of the progress being made, consider the needs of many people with physical disabilities who use personal computers to perform many important tasks. With the first popular machines, such as the Apple II, these people had to spend five to ten minutes changing disks every time they wanted to do something different. Today's operating systems, the programs that tell the computer what to do, are much easier for physically disabled people to manipulate. AT&T's UNIX™ operating system, for example, allows the user to perform several different tasks without changing disks. Digital Research, the company that gave us the CP/M® operating system, now sells an advanced program, called Concurrent DOS™, that permits multi-tasking; you can, for example, calculate some figures in one "window" and then, without changing disks, transfer those numbers to a report you are writing in another window. Microsoft, maker of MS-DOS™, is adding to its popular operating system a new program, called Windows™, that lets users view up to four different tasks at once. One critical advantage these new operating systems offer to physically disabled individuals: it is no longer necessary to re-enter information when you switch tasks. Today's operating systems allow data to be shared between, say, a word-processing program and a spreadsheet.

To illustrate how the powerful new personal computers and operating systems can help many persons with special needs, consider the problems facing an individual with severe cerebral palsy who uses a microcomputer to talk to others in the room as well as to write and to calculate. Cerebral palsy not only makes typing on a keyboard difficult, it also restricts speech. I walked into the office of a young professional with cerebral palsy last year. He was working on a spreadsheet program as I entered. To answer my question, he had to signal me to wait, conclude what he was doing, remove the disk from his computer, install a second disk, wait until it was ready for use, and then (a full five minutes later) type his answer to me.

Many of today's machines, including Apple's Macintosh and Lisa computers, AT&T's new 3B desktop computers, and other products using advanced operating systems, would let this man answer me with just two or three commands on the keyboard. Once we had finished our conversation, another two or three strikes on the keyboard would bring him back to where he was before we talked.

These capabilities were impossible for microcomputers to perform just a few years ago. Today, they're not only available but affordable. Apple's Macintosh, for example, sells for about the same price as does the 16-bit IBM PC. And the advanced operating systems often come with the computer or may be purchased separately at little extra cost.

Computer capabilities that cost $1 million in 1955 could be purchased in 1982 for around one 1955 dollar. This one fact helps to explain why such remarkable features in computers are so quickly becoming affordable to individuals and not just to businesses. By 1990 it probably will be possible to purchase circuitry one hundred times as powerful as the 1955 machines—for just one 1955 penny. It seems likely, then, that 32-bit machines will sell for what we are now accustomed to paying for less powerful machines. Indeed, InfoCorp, a Cupertino, California company specializing in computer market research, predicts that 32-bit computers will comprise 80 percent of all desktop models sold by 1990.

That does not mean, however, that the powerful new machines will do all they probably are capable of doing. Now, the frustrating compatibility problems are restricting such important functions as synthesized speech to a fraction of their actual potential. To resolve these difficulties and to forestall more problems in the near future, it is of vital importance that people with special needs communicate with hardware and software manufacturers to explain what they want to do and why existing products are inadequate to meet their needs.

America is now entering a new era, often called "The Information Age." In this country, as in many European nations, the ability to use microcomputers will soon be necessary for education, employment, shopping, banking, and many other aspects of daily living.

We entered an "Industrial Age" earlier in our history. It was not until almost the end of that era that it was possible for people with special needs to participate fully in our societies. In the U.S., accessibility in buildings and transportation systems did not command attention until the mid-1970s, when we discovered that we had erected government and private-sector buildings that many people with wheelchairs could not get into, transportation systems that many disabled people could not use, and telecommunications capabilities that were all but closed to millions of deaf people. Throughout Europe today, and in many American cities as well, accessibility remains more a goal than a reality. It has taken many laws, regulations, and civil-rights protests to get us to this point.

As we enter "The Information Age," we should realize that tens of millions of people will again be left behind if we do not act soon to ensure that they can gain access to information technologies. As other parts of the world, too, enter the computer era, which is happening quickly, as many as one-half billion people will be affected by the accessibility of information systems.

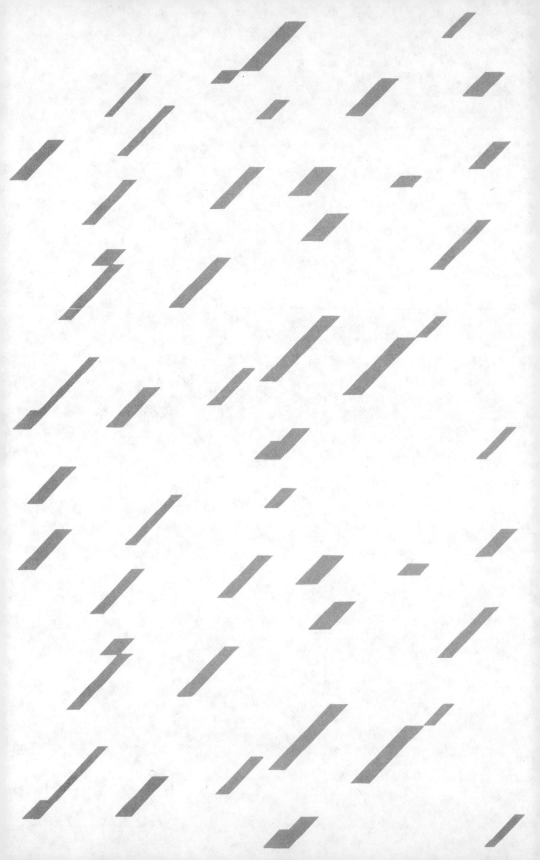

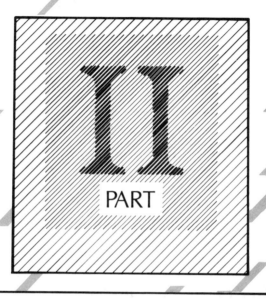

II

PART

MICROCOMPUTERS AND...

CHAPTER

3

EMPLOYMENT

"Do I like my work? I love it!"

In a small white house in the Fairfax Farms area of nothern Virginia, a man named Rick Pilgrim is doing things that, from a medical viewpoint, would be considered impossible for him to do. Ten years ago, when he was still a teenager, Rick was shot in a gun accident: "A friend of mine was sitting behind me, playing with this gun. I turned toward him. That's when the gun went off." The bullet entered Rick's spinal cord at nearly the base of his skull, causing an extremely severe spinal-cord injury that left him unable to move anything except his eyes and mouth. As he himself acknowledged: "C-1 quads [a medical term] don't usually survive."

Rick's arms, torso, and legs are still paralyzed, and he spends virtually all of his time in bed at home. As we talked, I noticed that he could not even move his neck.

The accident paralyzed his body, but it didn't hurt his mind or his sense of determination. He spent ten weeks in intensive care at a local hospital, followed by eleven months at a spinal-cord injury center. Returning home, Rick didn't waste any time getting his high-school equivalency diploma. And then he started working with computers.

In January 1976, with help from the state vocational rehabilitation agency and George Washington University's Job Development Laboratory, Rick learned about the Voice Data Entry System™ produced by small Scope Electronics. He spent two years in training, some of it conducted by Scope, learning how to use the technology to write programs in the FORTRAN and COBOL languages. By early 1978, he had written and documented his own inventory control system, all by voice.

The U.S. National Institutes of Health (NIH) hired Rick as a computer assistant in July of that year. Starting at four hours daily, he now works five hours each day, five days a week, and is shooting for a full 40-hour week. As his eyes meet yours, you know he intends to get there.

Scope Electronics, meanwhile, was purchased by Interstate Electronics Corporation. Interstate, based in Anaheim, California, sells about one hundred voice-entry systems a month. Most are bought by corporations and hospitals. The company claims that productivity by factory inspectors, who can use its products to make notes during inspections while keeping both hands free, may rise as much as 60 percent over that of inspectors using more traditional note-taking techniques. In hospitals, Interstate says, patients may order as many as 10,000 services by using an 80-word voice input vocabulary.

However, it is difficult to imagine applications of the technology more dramatic than those that occur every working day in the white house in Fairfax Farms. Rick's mother Inez turns on the Data General Nova 3™ terminal ("That's all I do," she says). The minicomputer, which readers may recall from Tracy Kidder's excellent book, *The Soul of a New Machine*, retains in memory "templates" which store imprints of Rick's voice pronouncing frequently used words.

When he sees "system ready" appear on the screen, Rick starts his work. Relying now on complete words ("random," "sequential," "space," and the like) and then on spelled-out words ("dear", for example, might be spelled: "Delta. Easy. Alpha. Romeo."), Rick performs his programming, as shown in Figure 3.1. The system understands, Rick says, some 90 to 95 percent of what he says. "Outside noise throws it off," he acknowledges.

Although co-workers at NIH describe his work as "outstanding," Rick remains convinced he can do more. A documentation and systems analysis specialist, he is determined to master yet more complex computer functions.

Even as I ask it, I know the question's answer. "Do I like my work?" Rick repeats. "I love it!"

The technology that makes it possible for Rick to use his mind to support himself in fulfilling employment is still at a fairly primitive stage of development. The Voice Data Entry System Rick uses is, he says, "a dinosaur." Today, Interstate Electronics offers a range of voice recognition products far superior to the "old" one Rick uses. Some of the Interstate components recognize eight different words, some as many as 200, with up to 99 percent accuracy.

The VRC008, for example, recognizes speech by detecting significant parameters in the spoken word or phrase, compares these

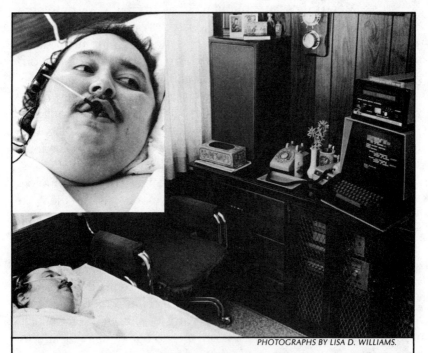

PHOTOGRAPHS BY LISA D. WILLIAMS.

Figure 3.1: *Rick Pilgrim documenting a computer program by voice. The Voice Data Entry System is on top of a Telray terminal. Inset, Rick wearing the Shure SM-10 headset, which contains the microphone he uses to talk to his computers.*

features with the stored sequences in its templates, and discards irrelevant information. The system then translates the recognized word into computer-understandable binary code, so that the machine "thinks" the word was entered by someone typing on its keyboard. The VRC is speaker-independent, meaning that it recognizes not only its primary user but other people as well. Designed for low-cost consumer products such as appliances, toys, games and other devices, it recognizes eight words or two-word commands (e.g., "channel four," "stop," etc.). The unit, which is actually a chip, is surprisingly inexpensive. A computer game manufacturer, for example, might purchase the units by the thousands at less than $10 each.

The more sophisticated VRT300, usable with DEC VT100 terminals and some CIT-101 models, recognizes a 100-word vocabulary with, the company says, 99 percent accuracy. It lists for about $1300.

Rick is aware of other new products—and these have him very excited. NIH has offered to provide him with an IBM PC. With this personal computer, Rick could use the PC-Mate Voice Recognition Board™ made by Tecmar, Inc. The $995 board uses 8K of memory to store up to 100 words; it can be upgraded to 200 words, for which it would require 16K of memory.

As I left Rick's house, I reflected on the remarkable difference between his attitude and that of so many quadriplegic and other severely disabled persons I've met in the U.S., Europe, and the Middle East. Rick, for one thing, is truly independent in the fullest sense of the word. He earns a salary that pays for his daily needs. On that salary, he pays federal, state, and local taxes. The investment made by the Virginia rehabilitation agency clearly has returned healthy dividends for the government. NIH's offer to install an IBM PC with voice-recognition capabilities illustrates that his employer, too, realizes that it gets more from Rick than it gives him.

Pure economics aside, what is most impressive about Rick Pilgrim is how satisfied the 29-year old is. His work gives his life purpose: "I'm fulfilled," he says.

I was reminded of the observations made by another quadriplegic man, Houston's Lex Frieden, on a recent trip to Europe. Lex's comments mirrored my own impressions. In Sweden and the Netherlands, Lex says, he and his wife Joyce met with several dozen severely disabled people, almost none of whom were employed:

> We discovered that there are more services and benefits for disabled people in both Sweden and the Netherlands than there are in the United States. In particular, income benefits and cash subsidies for disabled people are comparatively high in those countries. Both countries have a program for the centralized provision of and payment for technical aids and devices. These comprehensive systems not only provide aids, they prescribe, repair, evaluate, and replace those aids and devices as well. The aids are usually supplied free of charge by the government. They may include wheelchairs, elevators, remote control devices, automobiles, and so forth. Being poor is not a requirement for receiving assistance. We saw people using government-purchased wheelchairs which cost as much as $7,000 or $8,000. Additionally, the fewest number of wheelchairs that we found anyone having in Sweden was 7. We don't know what they did with them, but some people had as many as 20 wheelchairs that had been purchased for them by the government.
>
> Yet, in spite of these liberal benefits and extensive service networks, many of the disabled people we talked to were dissatisfied. They pointed out that many of the benefits they received discouraged independence and threatened motivation. Some of the people we talked to said they would like to go to work, but they couldn't afford to risk losing their benefits. Others said they had applied for jobs and been turned down because employers wanted to hire nondisabled people who needed the work because they did not have high pensions.

Rick Pilgrim received much less from government in America, and, through his taxes, he's already paid all of it back. More important, as he has discovered, work lends to life a sense of purpose and a degree of satisfaction no amount of government handouts can offer.

"I'm not feeling challenged enough"

Equally fulfilled is Kevin Riley. I talked with Kevin at his Silver Spring, Maryland, home while he was recovering from an illness.

The blue, aluminum-siding house features ramps he uses for his motorized wheelchair. At 31, Kevin is a programmer/analyst with IBM's Business Center in Bethesda, Maryland. He's worked for the company for six years, since completing his bachelor's degree at the University of Maryland in Russian and Chinese. ("Languages always have fascinated me," he says. "They're my first love.") Now he works with a different kind of language. Speaking about his work, he says: "We do all the business programming for IBM worldwide."

Kevin, like Rick, is a quadriplegic. In Kevin's case, the spinal-cord injury occurred in a motorcycle accident two years after he started working at IBM in a technical-support capacity. The company, which recognized his ability, retrained him in a more sedentary job in programming analysis. The adjustments were hard for Kevin to make. His life prior to the accident had been an active one, with frequent sporting activities, weight lifting, and other strenuous pursuits. With a serious spinal-cord injury, none of these remained possible for him.

Today, he uses a mouthstick to type on the IBM 3033 he uses at work and on the Apple microcomputer he has at home. His home unit is also equipped with Prentke Romich Environmental Control Unit (ECU™) peripherals that make it easier for him to control appliances and other devices in the house. For example, he can turn off all the lights in the house by pressing one switch. What excites him most, though, is the voice-controlled IBM PC he just got.

The Intel Electronics speech recognition unit equipped with a custom-made interface designed by George Markovsky, a White Plains IBM programmer assigned to the T. J. Watson Research Center, is capable of understanding 100 words in each of a theoretically unlimited number of data sets. Kevin could train each unit to recognize its full complement of words, using one unit for word processing, another for data processing, and the like. "It can go on forever," he says with a smile.

Kevin is also completing his law degree studies at Georgetown University: "I'm not feeling challenged enough," he explains. And he's started three small companies. One provides transportation for disabled people in the Maryland suburbs of Washington, D.C., a second does construction work, particularly additions to private homes, and a third handles a nursing registry. Kevin's rationale for these ventures is simple enough: in trying to meet his own needs, he's found a dearth of appropriate services in his geographical area. Besides, he adds, as long as he has to purchase vans, supervise alterations in his home to make it accessible, and arrange for his own medical care, he might as well turn these activities into profitable businesses.

The Prentke Romich Environmental Control Unit (ECU) technology is a diversified set of aids and devices designed to help people like Kevin maintain control over their environments. The pneumatic "puff-and-sip" mouthpiece he uses at his Bethesda office, for example, is distributed by Prentke Romich, which also supplies switches for control of intercoms, telephones, televisions, fans, and call signals. A BSR Command Module, which is commercially available through local hardware and computer stores, transmits the signals to telephone auto-dialers, radios, televisions, and other devices. As a result of these and similar peripherals, Kevin can juggle his many activities with minimal assistance from others. Without them, he could not work on one job, let alone fill his days as completely as he now does.

As Kevin's experience indicates, regaining control over one's personal life is vital for successful job seeking and working when one has a severe disability. The difference between working at home, as Rick Pilgrim does, and commuting to work and to school is a major one, involving difficult and time-consuming tasks. Kevin has to dress, eat, and transport himself to IBM's Bethesda offices as well as Georgetown's classrooms. The Prentke Romich and BSR devices make those tasks easier.

As important as the equipment is, the determination Kevin shares with Rick is much more critical to success in employment. Kevin shrugs off any comments on his remarkable sense of purpose. About his law-school studies, start-up companies, and work at IBM, he says merely: "They make life more interesting."

"This job would be impossible"

In Little Rock, Arkansas, Dennis Holzhauser, 35, works as a computer specialist at the Cooperative Extension Service of the Graduate Institute of Technology. Dennis uses a TRS-80 Model II computer equipped with four disk drives to write programs documenting how pesticides are used by Arkansas farmers.

Holzhauser, who is legally blind, has never been a farmer. His vision started deteriorating at 19: "It's either retinitis pigmentosa or something very much like it," he explains. Above the Model II screen is a mirror that reflects the image to a Visualtek™ camera. The camera, in turn, is attached to a second monitor, this one capable of displaying characters as high as four inches and as wide as three inches. Dennis can see those enlarged characters through his thick-lensed glasses.

To read books and other documents, Dennis uses a Voyager™ closed-circuit television monitor that also enlarges images. The Voyager is also made by Visualtek, a Santa Monica, California, company specializing in aids for blind individuals.

Dennis describes his job by talking about pesticides. "Let's say you're a farmer. You want to know what a given pesticide will do for you, what plants to use it with, and what insects to use it against. If something happens with the pesticide that you didn't expect, you need someone to call. That's me." He's had the job for almost two years now. "Before we wrote this program, you needed to spend hours researching a given pesticide's side effects. Now I can do that work in a minute." He writes his own programs and keys them into the computer. He likes the equipment so much he got a $2,000 Voyager to use at home to read his mail. It also helps him in the courses he is taking at the University of Arkansas at Little Rock.

Most of the equipment he uses at work was purchased by the state rehabilitation agency, the Office for the Blind and Visually Impaired. The Cooperative Extension Service, however, bought the Radio Shack Model II. The two Visualtek machines Dennis uses are quite expensive compared to the cost of the computer itself. Not many severely disabled individuals will be able to afford to spend as much as $2,000 just for one peripheral, especially on top of the $2,500 often needed to buy a microcomputer. This illustrates why it is so important that government agencies and private employers purchase the necessary special aids. But the cost associated with the Visualtek equipment is interesting for another reason. I've said earlier that aids marketed to the general public often are inexpensive because mass-production techniques can be used to drive down costs. The BSR Command Module that Kevin Riley uses, for example, costs just $40. Visualtek's products, by contrast, are made with the special needs of blind and low-vision people in mind. Accordingly, costs are much higher because there are relatively few blind individuals in this country. Are those high costs worth paying? For government and for industry, the answer is undoubtedly yes. Blind individuals capable of doing productive work contribute both to their employers and to government; denying these people the aids they need to work deprives both the employer and the government of their contributions.

Could he do his work without the computer and its peripherals? "This job would be impossible, Frank, without these aids. It would be extremely difficult and someone else would have to key in the programs I wrote, assuming I could write them."

Dennis, who doesn't know Braille, is enthusiastic about the potential of programming jobs for other individuals who are blind. "You need a logical mind," he says, adding: "If you can handle the frustration involved in this kind of work, your vision won't hurt you. It's important, though, to get the proper training and to have the right equipment." He himself came to Arkansas from Pennsylvania to take advantage of the computer-programming course offered by the Little Rock-based Arkansas Enterprises for the Blind. The nine-month program is a demanding one, requiring up to 60 hours of study each week; graduates learn as much as others do in a more leisurely two-year curriculum. An added advantage of attendance at the Arkansas Enterprises for the Blind program was unexpected: it was there that he met his wife, Diana, who is also blind.

The next day, I visited the 32-year old, brown-haired Diana in her office at the State Employment Security Division. When I saw her computer programming equipment, I asked the obvious question. "Well, when Dennis got interested, I did, too. I guess that explains it," she said with a laugh.

Diana was born blind in Pearland, Texas, a small (pop. 10,000) town near Houston. She went to the University of Texas in Austin for a bachelor's degree in music and a master's in voice pedagogy, hoping to teach singing. "It was hard to get a job, though. The most I could manage in Austin was a part-time position. So I decided to come to Little Rock, hoping for a job in communication services work, perhaps with blind people." When she learned that most jobs in human-services fields require an educational background different from her own, however, she became more amenable to considering a different line of work.

When I expressed surprise that a music lover would like programming, she told me: "You'd be surprised! Music is closer to programming than you think. There's sequencing, detail work. A lot of music majors are going into programming these days, and liking it."

Unlike her husband, Diana has no usable vision. So she relies in her work as a computer programmer on an Optacon™ reading system manufactured by Telesensory Systems of Palo Alto, California. The Optacon is equipped with a lens for reading cathode-ray tubes (CRTs), such as computer monitor screens. The $2,275 device (the lens is an additonal $375) produces a tactile output of raised images on a small (1" by 1½") array. Diana uses her index finger to sense the vibrating signal instead of trying to read the computer terminal screen. She types information on the keyboard and then uses the Optacon to read it back; her behavior is exactly the same as that of any other computer programmer, except that she uses a different sense to verify what she has done. In this way, she uses the device much as Stephen Rogers uses his speech synthesizer: to translate information from a medium that is not helpful to one that is. Diana likes the Optacon: "It's worked out surprisingly well." With it, she's produced seventeen programs in six months. "I did one program in just three days. My supervisor said it would have taken most programmers a week or more to do the same job."

The Optacon requires considerable training; interpreting the tactile signals is something that takes time, just as synthesized speech usually requires some getting used to, as Dr. Rogers discovered. Equally helpful on the job, but easier to learn, is Versabraille™, a portable Braille and audio information system marketed by Telesensory Systems. The $7,000 device (including cable) can store on tape as many as 400 pages of material in Braille. And, unlike many Braille-based devices, it is small and easily portable. As illustrated in Figure 3.2, Diana uses the Versabraille for note taking and other programming work.

I asked her about her job-seeking experiences. Did the availability of the equipment make a difference for her? "Oh, yes, I'm quite sure it did," she answered:

> Unfortunately, most people still think blind persons are beggars. And most, sadly, have absolutely no idea what we can do with

today's machines. I took samples of my work at Arkansas Enterprises for the Blind with me on job interviews, together with brochures about the equipment that I was trained to use. A lot of people were truly impressed. It's just amazing. When I got the job offer, the state rehabilitation agency purchased the special equipment I needed. There's no question that my employment interviewer had a better appreciation of my potential after he learned of the equipment I would bring with me to this job.

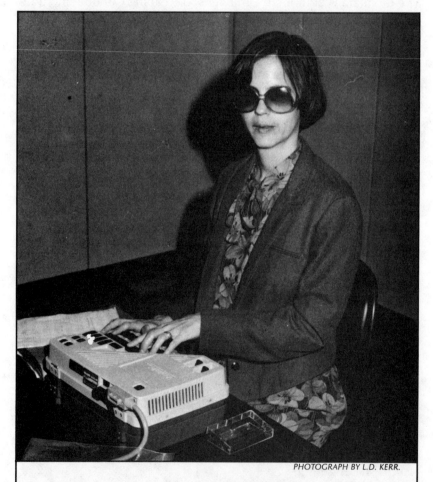

PHOTOGRAPH BY L.D. KERR.

Figure 3.2: Diana Holzhauser takes notes using her Versabraille machine.

"It becomes very gratifying"

Michael Dickman, of Brooklyn, New York, whose legs were paralyzed by polio, didn't need a computer to show anybody how he could do his work. He needed it to keep up with a mushrooming work load. The tax law practice he had founded ten years ago was growing so fast he couldn't keep up, even with two full-time assistants. So Dickman, who got his two degrees in law from New York University, bought a Vector Graphics small computer in 1980. "I chose the Vector because it ran the software I wanted," Dickman said, giving advice anyone would be wise to follow. Quick Tax, Inc., a small Staten Island, New York, firm, produced Quick Tax, a program for tax preparers.

Soon, he added another computer. WordStar, a word-processing package he needed to correspond with his ever-growing list of clients, was the next addition. In 1983, he picked up an accounting package to help with his work for business clients.

Dickman is an example of a disabled person who uses computers but who does not require special adaptations to benefit from them. He is sole proprietor of a tax law practice that works with many disabled people as well as many low-income people: "I want to help others, Frank, I get satisfaction knowing that I'm doing something helpful. It becomes very gratifying."

Would he recommend tax law to other ambitious disabled people? "The law is a very great asset, but it is also very demanding. If you're willing to study, very hard and for a very long time, it's worth it. But you can do taxes without a law degree. Tax preparation might be a good career for someone who is good with numbers."

Mike uses crutches to walk up one flight of steep stairs to reach his office. There he settles into a wheelchair for the day. When I ask him why he doesn't take some of the profits from his proprietorship and get a ground-floor office, his answer reveals the businessman in the man: "This is convenient for my clients, Frank. Besides, the rent is low!"

But the computers he wouldn't give up for mere money. "I couldn't possibly do without these machines. There's absolutely no question that they've helped me keep up with the work load."

"When the system is up, I'm up!"

Also using two computers, but for different reasons, is Michael Ward, a program specialist with Special Education Programs, a division of the U.S. Department of Education in Washington, D.C. Mike's system features one Apple IIe that runs his programs and a second Apple that serves as his input station (Figure 3.3). The two are connected by cable; hard disks provide storage. Mike, whose cerebral palsy makes his speech difficult to understand, uses an Apple computer to communicate with people as well as to write reports. He speaks slowly in a voice that is readily intelligible to

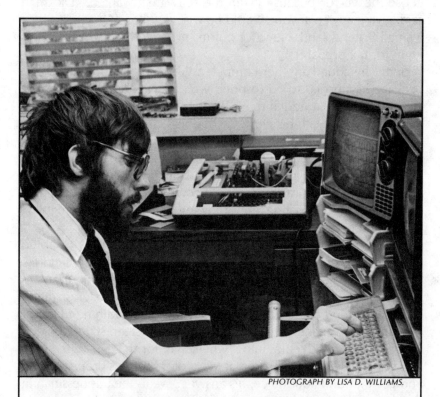

PHOTOGRAPH BY LISA D. WILLIAMS.

Figure 3.3: Mike Ward hits the keys of one Apple computer, which runs his "menu" program. Once Mike is satisfied with his text, he sends the information to the second Apple, which contains his word-processing program. Notice the unused keyboard at the rear. The system makes the second Apple "think" the commands are coming from that keyboard.

people who know him well but hard to follow for others. Mike uses a "menu" of words and phrases he can call up to the computer screen with one or a few keystrokes. Because one question he's often asked by visitors is, "How do you use these machines?" Mike has prepared an elaborate answer that he can display with two quick keystrokes.

Cerebral palsy also makes his finger movements erratic. To keep from striking the wrong keys, Mike has a keyboard guard that fits over the Apple IIe computer's keyboard. The guard helps him restrain his finger movements, so that only the correct keys (and not neighboring keys) are hit. The same disability makes Mike a slower-than-average typist. To overcome the speed problem, Mike uses a special routine that allows him to type one or two letters instead of an entire word; it is the same menu he uses for personal communication with visitors. Once Mike has selected the words and phrases he wants, he can send them to the second Apple computer on his desk, which holds his word-processing program.

In effect, the system makes the other Apple "think" that the information is being typed on its keyboard. At first, the use of two full-feature computers seems needlessly extravagant, until you realize that Mike could not run his menu program and the word-processing program on the same machine. If he were restricted to just one Apple, Mike would spend inordinate amounts of time entering one letter at a time; with the two computers, he increases his output by a factor of three or more.

Mike is very pleased with his system. "I love it!" he exclaims, pointing out that it makes him more productive than he has been in three decades: "When the system is 'up,' I'm 'up'; when it's 'down,' I'm 'down'!" He has learned BASIC, a programming language, and is now using it to write his own programs.

Gregg Vanderheiden, the University of Wisconsin computer-aids specialist who designed Mike's system, heads the Trace Research and Development Center, an important site of activity in the special-communication aids fields. Vanderheiden points out that the major problem Mike Ward faced was one of communication speed: "It turns out that rate is much more important than form for conversation, that is, whether it is visual or vocal. Normal conversation takes place at the rate of about 180 words per minute. Conversation can be held at slower rates, but it is extremely difficult to carry on a conversation in the usual sense of the word if the communication rate is limited to

Mike's 20 or so words per minute." The same is true in writing. For Mike Ward, working as he does in a federal bureaucracy, handling large amounts of paperwork and generating timely reports are essential to his job. The two computers, together with the message-option display, let him keep up with the demanding pace of his colleagues in his work.

Mike obviously is sometimes frustrated by the fact that his mind works much faster than do his communication capabilities. It is possible, some day, notes Paul Anderek, a computer-instruction specialist with the Department of Education, that Mike might want to use a speech synthesizer to speed up his conversation. Today's artificial voices are not yet clear enough for this purpose; some wags say the synthesizers speak with an "American computer accent." But, for Mike and many other persons with severe cerebral palsy, an improved unit may someday speak quickly and clearly.

It is not something Mike Ward feels he needs right now. The system he has offers him so dramatically great an enhancement in communication that he is more than delighted with what he can do now. It is easy for the observer to understand why. Only in his office, with his system, can he approach in volume of work anything resembling his potential; more primitive tools are extremely slow, sometimes maddeningly so. Perhaps that's one of the greatest potential benefits of microcomputers: to let people do more of what they're capable of doing.

"It's a natural for deaf people"

Tommy Walker, who is deaf, has been a printer with the Arkansas *Gazette* in Little Rock for 12 years. By preference, he works the night shift. During the day, with the help of his Franklin 1000™ personal computer, Tommy handles a small printing business of his own. The computer, which he bought because it was "Apple-compatible" yet less expensive than an Apple, is equipped with word- and data-processing software he uses to keep the books on his business, prepare his tax returns, and handle business correspondence. He also uses the machine to keep mailing lists for several organizations of deaf people in the central Arkansas area. "A computer is good for the deaf," he points out. "You don't have to be able to hear to use it."

It is clearly a machine he enjoys. "Sometimes I'll sit down here at 10:30 in the morning. The next time I look up, the sun is setting." His daughters Connie, 15, and Carrie, 10, use it for games and instructional purposes. "Connie learned how to type by working with this computer. In her first year, she's already up to 40 words per minute," Walker says, with a father's understandable pride.

Tommy, a long-time leader in the Arkansas deaf community, is concerned that deaf people may not be joining the "computer revolution" fast enough. He sees others around him using personal computers, but so far as he knows he's the only deaf person in the area to have one. "You don't have to be an expert to use this, Frank. And it's a natural for deaf people. By using a modem, you can communicate with hearing people who have computers as well as with deaf people who have TDDs [Telecommunications Devices for the Deaf, portable machines that allow deaf people to type instead of talk when using the telephone]. It's clearly the coming thing these days."

With the exception of some auditory signals and other sounds computer hardware and software sometimes make, Walker is right about computers being accessible to deaf people for employment, educational, and recreational uses. Writing about computer games in *High Technology*, Herb Brody observes: "Most video games could be played by a deaf person." He means the comment to be disparaging; he wants games designers to make better use of the computer's sound-generation capabilities: "The sound effects—mostly computerish beep-boop music and amplified static 'explosions'—convey no information needed to play the game."

With word-processing, accounting, and other general interest programs all available to him, Walker doesn't have to worry about expensive peripherals and their compatibility problems. Ultimately, it should be possible for people with other kinds of disabilities to use personal computers "off the shelf" with few, if any special adaptations. Reaching that stage will propel many thousands more disabled adults into productive and satisfying employment.

The Impact of Employment

Perhaps the single most remarkable thing about the people we've seen using microcomputers at work is how dynamic, how active, and how determined they seem to be. Indeed, it is difficult, if not impossible, to reconcile these profiles with the stereotypical image that Diana Holzhauser refers to when she says that "most people think blind persons are beggars." Recalling what Lex Frieden said about the pervasive sense of unhappiness among many European individuals who received large governmental handouts but had to take, along with these benefits, restrictions on their activities, particularly with respect to work, it is clear that there is something about challenging work that brings out the best in most of us, that transforms our lives into ever-greater assaults on preconceived notions of what is possible.

It may be that one of the magical aspects of microcomputers is that they free people from the shackles of disability, enabling them to live their lives based, not on what they cannot do, but on what they can do. Look, for example, at Mike Ward. The frustration of struggling daily against a disability that slows his communication to a snail's pace is so great that he could hardly be faulted for despairing of ever reaching his potential. The personal computer offers Mike the chance to do three times as much work as he used to do without it. Suddenly, Mike feels much more alive—and tremendously excited.

Or consider Rick Pilgrim. Until he was in his late teens, Rick found little challenging about his life; in fact, he dropped out of high school. That he was intelligent was evident from early childhood, but it seemed that something was missing. The gun accident happened, then, to someone that few people would refer to as a compulsive overachiever. Yet, when offered the chance to do competitive work using microcomputers, Rick was able to surmount even his severe spinal cord injury and to drive himself to heights his doctors never expected him to reach.

I would argue that Rick is immeasurably more alive, more self-actualized (to use Abraham Maslow's term), and yes, more fulfilled as a quadriplegic than he was as an able-bodied teen—or than many people with less severe disabilities are today. The major difference, it seems, is not so much the computer itself as what it allowed Rick to do. It released him from bondage, from dependence on others, and from the mind-bending boredom of empty days.

Like Rick, Kevin Riley probably works much more now than he did prior to his accident; certainly, it was only after the motorcycle severed his spinal cord that he started law school, set up three small companies, and also worked full time. Again, it is not so much that the computer does something for him as that it allows *him* to do something. These activities, in turn, become rewarding in themselves, far more in fact than the activites pursued by many of the disabled beneficiaries Lex Frieden met in Sweden.

These brief portraits also show some of the ways that severely disabled people have been able to obtain the aids they now use. In Rick's case, the state rehabilitation agency supplied him with much of the equipment he needed in order to be trained as a programmer. That, as I've mentioned several times already, is a good investment for government to make, because, by working, Rick will be paying taxes, not receiving benefits supported by the taxes of others.

Federal and state legislation enable state vocational rehabilitation agencies to purchase for severely disabled persons those aids and devices that appear needed in order for the individual to be trained for, or to accept, gainful employment. Although criteria vary somewhat from state to state, in general, an individual must have a medical condition that is expected to last at least six months and that prohibits or limits employment. When such a device could make the difference between working and not working, state rehabilitation agencies often will pick up at least part of the costs of the aid. At times, as when the disabled individual has substantial personal resources, the state and the individual may split the expense; at other times, the person's employer may share in the costs with the state agency.

For the address of your state agency, contact the Council of State Administrators of Vocational Rehabilitation (1055 Thomas Jefferson St., NW, Washington, DC 20007).

For disabled individuals whose limitations are service-connected, the Veterans Administration (VA) may purchase needed aids and devices. Indeed, the VA is somewhat more generous on behalf of veterans than state rehabilitation agenices are with civilians, primarily because of more liberal legislation and relatively more available funds. An excellent source of information about the programs is the VA itself (write: Veterans Administration, Washington, DC 20420). And don't forget the outstanding service organization, the Disabled American Veterans (DAV). The DAV can help you cut through "red tape" and get appropriate action from the VA quickly. DAV maintains a Washington, DC office for exactly this reason, among others. (Write: Disabled American Veterans, National Service and Legislative Headquarters, 807 Maine Ave., SW, Washington, DC 20024.)

Both state rehabilitation agencies and the VA have the authority to pay all or part of the costs of aids and devices needed by a disabled individual who desires to move to a better, higher-paying job. Thus, it is not necessary for the individual to be unemployed in order to qualify for assistance with the cost of microcomputers or other accommodation aids. However, in recent years, budgetary constraints have limited support for those already employed. As Kevin's story illustrates, doing good work for an employer may result in the company providing needed equipment. We saw this, too, with Rick, when NIH secured for him an IBM PC.

Some private employers, particularly larger ones, are subject to two little-known federal laws: section 402 of the 1974 Vietnam era Veterans Readjustment Assistance Act and section 503 of the 1973 Rehabilitation Act. Section 402 contains provisions ensuring disabled veterans and veterans of the Vietnam era of certain civil rights in employment. Private firms doing business with the federal government are subject to the requirements of section 402 to the extent that their contracts in any given year exceed the rather nominal sum of $10,000. The language appearing in the regulations implementing section 402 also appears, almost word for word, in regulations written to put into effect section 503 of the 1973 Rehabilitation Act. Section 503 applies to businesses holding more than $2,500 in federal contacts. Both sections are administered by the U.S. Department of Labor.

Both sections contain provisions forbidding overt discrimination on the basis of disability and the requirement that the contractor provide, on behalf of disabled applicants and employees, what are called "reasonable accommodations." The term is not defined in either set of rules, but examples are given to illustrate what is meant; helpful too, is a long series of judicial interpretations. Today, we understand a "reasonable" accommodation to be one that is needed by a disabled person to perform a job for which the individual is qualified and that does not impose an "undue hardship" upon the contractor. That is, when an applicant or employee is qualified for a particular job (meets the criteria for employment) but needs some aid or other kind of assistance in order to do that job, the contractor is obligated by federal law to consider the purchase or lease of such an accommodation. The company has the option of declining to obtain the aid on the grounds that to do so would impose an undue hardship on the business (usually: would cost too much or would subject employees to unnecessary danger), but the regulations for sections 402 and 503 allow the individual to appeal an adverse decision.

The importance of the requirement that large businesses doing contract work for federal agencies provide "reasonable" accommodations is that, as I have shown, such aids may indeed make the difference between working well and working poorly. Suppose, for purposes of illustration, Company A advertises for an accounting position. Were a fully qualified and trained accountant to apply for that job, the company (if it is a federal contractor) could not refuse to hire the individual merely because she or he had a disability. Nor could Company A reject the applicant on the grounds that an accommodation would be necessary. Rather, the firm must grant to this person fair and objective consideration for employment. If it finds the individual to be the best qualified applicant, it must consider ways to provide "reasonable accommodations" to meet the candidate's particular disability-related needs.

Company B, to continue with our illustration, has an opening for a chemical engineer. Were a disabled person not qualified to do that work to apply for the job, could the company refuse to employ the applicant? Of course, the answer is yes: the applicant did not qualify for the job. Sections 402 and 503 protect only *qualified* disabled job applicants and employees.

One other major piece of legislation provides for employers to pay for accommodation aids and other kinds of help that qualified disabled persons need. This is section 504, following section 503 in the 1973 Rehabilitation Act. Section 504 offers similar accommodation privileges to disabled persons. A series of judicial interpretations has established that section 504 does apply to employment. However, the statute does not apply to federal contractors, but instead to recipients of federal grants. Colleges, universities, vocational-technical schools, libraries, social service agencies, hospitals, and the like are required to make their programs accessible to and usable by persons with disabilities.

Section 504 is a powerful ally for handicapped individuals seeking job training and employment. To learn more about this statute, which is often called "the bill of rights for handicapped people," contact the offices for civil rights in the federal Department of Education, Department of Health and Human Services, and the Department of Labor (Office for Civil Rights, USED, Washington, DC 20202; Office for Civil Rights, USHHS, Washington, DC 20201; and Office of Federal Contract Compliance Programs, USDOL, Washington, DC 20201). Other good sources of information are listed in this book, including Project HEATH (Higher Education and the Handicapped), the Disabled American Veterans, and the National Center for a Barrier Free Environment.

Not all private employers are covered by sections 402, 503, and 504. The first two (sections 402 and 503) apply only to federal contractors and subcontractors, of which there are a few hundred thousand in the U.S. Few private businesses are subject to section 504, but most education, health, and social service agencies at the federal and state levels of governments are required to comply with its provisions. The vast bulk of employers in the nation, however, are small or medium-sized firms that do no grant or contract work for any unit of government; they may be required by state or local laws to practice nondiscrimination toward disabled persons who have special needs. Thirty-nine states have such laws. To find out what laws affect employers in your area, contact the President's Committee on Employment of the Handicapped (1111 Twentieth St., NW, Washington, DC 20036), who will probably refer you to a governor's committee or perhaps to a mayor's committee that can answer your questions with up-to-date information.

Employer Awareness

Persons who are disabled often know from long experience that few employers are sophisticated enough to recognize their abilities behind the smokescreen presented by obvious and severe disabilities. Indeed, tens of millions of handicapped individuals have given up hope of finding gainful employment commensurate with their abilities and training. There are signs, however, that important progress is being made.

Not surprisingly, much of the leadership in the private sector is being assumed by financial services, electronics, and telecommunications companies. These firms not only are among the fastest growing in the country but also offer employment that in many cases requires less in the way of "Greek god" physical perfection than do most jobs in traditional industries. Contrast, for example, the work of an assembly-line employee at General Motors with that of a computer programmer. The GM worker stands for hours on end, reacting quickly to the ever-moving line, using both hearing and vision to coordinate movements to the requirements of the assembly process. A programmer need not stand at all. Speed of hand-eye coordination is much less critical than is trained judgment. And the programmer has available sophisticated equipment, including the computer itself, to help with the work. Little hearing or lifting is required.

To illustrate, consider some innovations at American Express, the financial services company headquartered in lower Manhattan. According to James Raney, the firm's senior vice president for banking operations, American Express began to employ severely disabled persons as word-processing staff members in 1982. These new employees worked in their homes, not in company offices. American Express installed Wang and Lanier word-processing equipment in their homes, contracted for the installation of three to four telephone lines connecting the worker with the company's central offices, and placed safety and health equipment, such as fire extinguishers, in work locations to satisfy Occupational Safety and Health Administration (OSHA) requirements. In doing all of this, American Express was exceeding the requirements of federal law for "reasonable accommodations." Not every company could afford to make the investments American Express made, but perhaps that's the point: financial services corporations, much like electronics and telecommunications businesses, can offer employment opportunities for people whose severe disabilities present problems that other kinds of companies cannot resolve.

By early 1984 the "electronic cottage" approach to the employment of home-based individuals at American Express was ready to expand from the initial group of ten employees. Raney comments that it was actually less expensive for the company to install the equipment in the workers' homes than to rent office space in Manhattan. The employees' work is monitored by supervisors who review the work they produce and transmit over telephone lines to the office word-processing equipment. The firm is able to supervise the workers without having to see them, and the employees' work hours are tracked electronically. They work 35-hour weeks, selecting their own hours.

New York Telephone has several workers who use the same electronic-cottage approach for different reasons. In one instance, both husband and wife work for the company. To take care of their preschool child, they stagger their work hours so that at least one of them is always with the child. Because their computer equipment is connected with the company's office terminals, they only need to commute from Long Island to Manhattan one or two days a week.

In Little Rock, Arkansas, Jack McSpadden is using computer equipment to keep up with the huge amounts of paperwork required by his job and by his civic activities. A recruiter for Southwestern Bell, Jack also serves as a member of a federal agency board. His board position requires that he read some eight hundred pages of technical material each year. Jack is blind. In years past, he would have asked his assistant to read the voluminous material to him. But Jack's employer has provided him with sophisticated "talking" computer equipment and has installed computer peripherals that enable Jack to read in Braille whatever is typed into word processors in the agency's Washington office.

In Murray Hill, New Jersey, AT&T Bell Laboratories has provided several blind research scientists with equipment similar to McSpadden's. And, as mentioned, for Kevin Riley IBM has supplied advanced technology to allow a valued employee to transfer to a new job after a motorcycle accident. Manufacturers Hanover Trust considers speech-output computers to be an "ordinary and necessary" part of its employment program, according to human resources analyst John Reid.

Sometimes the employment of disabled persons occurs from dire necessity. Equitable Life's national benefits section employs 4,000 persons in ten work locations nationwide to pay more than $2.5 million in claims each year. The work involves processing as many as twenty million pieces of paper annually. Once a backlog develops, says Edward Corton, division vice president, it has a "snowball" effect: "You receive a lot of inquiries from claimants, and this in turn slows the processing of claims even more." Such a backlog developed in 1982. Searching for help, Equitable hit on the idea of "farming out" some of the claims-processing work to nontraditional workers. In California, the company turned to housewives and retired individuals, supplying them with computer terminals and the necessary training. The program worked well. When a similar backlog appeared in the Northeast, Equitable was confident about its farming-out concept and turned to a group of eight severely handicapped persons who did the work at a Long Island–based rehabilitation facility. Seven of the eight are still in the program, producing quality work quickly, and the company has eliminated the backlog.

Sometimes the move to employ disabled persons arises from a long-established corporate commitment to hiring persons with special needs. DuPont is one company that has been a national leader for almost two decades in employing handicapped individuals. The Delaware firm is particularly interested in keeping older workers who become disabled through illness or accident. As far back as 1972, DuPont encouraged a computer programmer who became blind because of a tumor to return to work after just three months of medical rehabilitation. The company helped him learn Braille, bought an Optacon for him to use, and kept him on the job. Much as Diana Holzhauser does in Little Rock, he uses Braille and the Optacon to program on his computer. In 1978 a second DuPont worker developed multiple sclerosis, a severe and often progressive disorder that weakened his arm and leg muscles. The company got him a special "light-touch" computer to make it easier for him to type his reports. A short time later, DuPont was puzzled when an applicant with a strong work history repeatedly failed simple written tests. Exploring the situation with the help of outside consultants, DuPont discovered that the individual had dyslexia. The test was administered again, this time orally. The individual passed and now has been at work successfully for more than six years.

To appreciate what happened at DuPont, consider that in 1972 there were no federal laws requiring affirmative action on behalf of disabled persons. To use computer equipment to make accommodations for disabled employees was, at the time, revolutionary: it demolished the myth of a "barrier." DuPont demonstrated that severely disabled persons could return to productive employment using computer technology. The company's success in this area was one of the critical events that eventually convinced the U.S. Congress that affirmative action on behalf of disabled individuals was a realistic goal. And DuPont hasn't stopped there. As of 1983, the number of disabled employees at DuPont had increased more than 50 percent over the already high level it had achieved in 1972.

The European Experience

The use of microcomputers in Europe, particularly in Germany, is rapidly increasing. France has produced some of the best training programs for introducing novices to the wonders of the personal computer, and Sweden has demonstrated the power of the computer in managing a complex welfare state. However, the virtual absence of applications of the personal computer to enable disabled persons to work is striking. Even more disconcerting, to me at least, is a more fundamental difference between the American and European attitudes. While at least some governmental and private programs in the U.S. are based on the concept that many persons with special needs can and should work, in England, the Scandinavian countries, and many other European nations, I sometimes found sheer incomprehension when I began talking about putting special-needs persons to work in plants and offices.

This problem seems to have little to do with computers. Rather, the tradition of governmental care for persons who have disabilities is so powerful in most of Europe that it overwhelms advances in technology. Earlier in this chapter, my friend Lex Frieden demonstrated the pervasive "we will take care of you because you cannot care for yourself" mentality in Europe—and showed how devastating such paternalism can be for people who seek to show that they are more able than disabled. Before much of Europe awakens to the potential of the microcomputer in employment of persons with special needs, the more prosaic idea that these people can work at all must surface.

Ironically, economics may prove to be the key that turns this ancient lock. In the United Kingdom, the social bureaucracy dispensing governmental benefits for disabled and older persons has become so obfuscated and complex that not even the "experts" know for sure who is entitled to what under which circumstances. The welfare machinery seems to work more smoothly in Sweden, yet there, as in England, the cost of maintaining huge numbers of older and disabled individuals on public aid rolls is menacing the integrity of the state economy. As we have seen most clearly with Rick Pilgrim, helping someone to support himself is much less costly to government than is maintaining that person on public assistance programs for life.

As the costs of microcomputer technologies fall, and they soon will, such people as England's George Wilson and France's Anders Arnor, both experts on the employment of persons with special needs, will be able to penetrate the social-welfare mentality so pervasive throughout Europe today. International companies, such as ITT, IBM, and AT&T International, will transport their knowledge and technologies to Europe to keep on the job employees who become disabled. These innovations may have as dramatic an effect in Europe as DuPont's experimental approaches had in the U.S. in 1972.

Another effect I anticipate is a decentralization of the employment of persons with special needs. In Japan, particularly, but in England as well, the disabled persons who do work tend to be employed in "special" firms rather than in the general workplace. The United Kingdom's Remploy, for example, does contract work for governmental and private clients, operating much as do "sheltered workshops" in the U.S. Nine of every ten Remploy workers are disabled. Microcomputer technology permits much greater employment of persons with special needs in the same offices, plants, and stores where nondisabled persons work. This idea, which I confess sounds elementary, is more a dream than a reality in most of the world, and, lest I sound too chauvinistic, I must add that the U.S. also has a whole host of sheltered workshops. Here, as elsewhere, the notion that people with disabilities are people with abilities has yet to take firm hold in the public mind.

It Can Be Done

Perhaps nothing is more important, with respect to the employment of older and disabled persons, than to demonstrate that it can be done. AT&T is an example of a major corporation that has shown that employment of qualified disabled individuals helps both those people and the company. The communications giant is one of

America's leading employers in the area of affirmative action for handicapped individuals and disabled veterans. AT&T's experience is mirrored by that of DuPont, IBM, and American Express.

Perhaps that's the best ally disabled persons seeking work could ask for: armed with the knowledge that popular myths about their inability to be productive employees are often false, together with information about computer-based aids and devices that are available to help them, these jobseekers can approach employers with confidence.

As Diana Holzhauser's success reminds us, disabled applicants are well advised not to assume that prospective employers understand that modern technology can provide inexpensive and reasonable accommodation. Taking a leaf from her book, job seekers could bring with them to the employment interview brochures and other brief explanations of how specific devices could be used on the job. Such materials can help the applicant answer the interviewer's questions about how he or she could perform the work.

Information about precedents in the employment of handicapped persons may be obtained by writing to the President's Committee on Employment of the Handicapped (address given earlier). For additional information about job-related accommodation aids and devices, two publications are particularly helpful: my own *Reasonable Accommodation Handbook,* originally published by AT&T and now distributed by the National Center for a Barrier Free Environment (1015 Fifteenth St., NW, Washington, DC 20005), and *Directory of Living Aids for the Disabled Person,* published by the Veterans Administration, and available from the U.S. Government Printing Office (Washington, DC 20402).

Job applicants can also tell employers about the Job Accommodation Network (JAN), which is jointly sponsored by the President's Committee on Employment of the Handicapped and the University of West Virginia. Employers interested in learning more about available aids and devices may call the committee on the toll-free number 1-800-JAN-PCEH to receive up-to-date computerized information on the features, prices, and availability of many hundreds of accommodations.

However, the dominant impression I received from talking with Rick Pilgrim, Kevin Riley, Dennis and Diana Holzhauser, Tommy Walker, Mike Dickman, Mike Ward, Jack McSpadden, and others has nothing to do with microcomputers or other aids and devices. These people got jobs and kept them *because they had something to offer.* Some knew tax law, printing, employment processes, or special education programming, and some knew computers. Their employers hired them to take advantage of their special skills and knowledge.

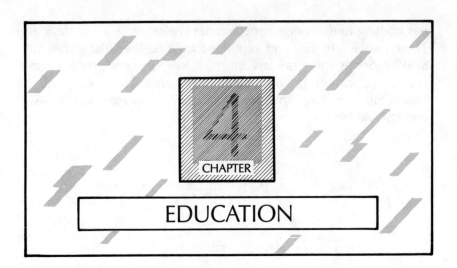

CHAPTER 4

EDUCATION

In a resource room in Fairbanks, Alaska, learning-disabled students are doing some things long-time teacher Nancy Sopp thought she'd never see. They're coming to school early and leaving late. They're teaching each other. And they're teaching gifted children who also use the resource room how to program computers. Sopp reports that some students, whose handwritten compositions seemed to demonstrate near illiteracy, "suddenly possessed the ability to write complete sentences. They care about spelling. They stomp up to me (we wear big boots here) as the snow forms a puddle and the tardy bell rings to announce that they've been thinking about some changes they want to make in their LOGO procedures."

Sopp's junior high school students use Broderbund's Bank Street Writer™ word-processing program on an Apple II Plus personal computer to write class reports, creative-writing assignments, and notes to pen pals. "Many of my students are poor readers and can't begin to read the instructions in the manual or tutorial," Sopp reports. They can, however, learn to read the menu lists and other function words on the computer screen. One student, Sopp says, displays some autistic behavior and is classified as educable mentally retarded. "He possesses a phenomenal amount of information about airlines," she reports. Tapping this interest, through the PFS:® FILE program published by Software Publishing Corporation, she was able to help him set up his own information storage and retrieval system containing information about which airlines fly which routes.

As Sopp's experience in Fairbanks illustrates, special educators need not restrict themselves to "special" equipment and software. Often, off-the-shelf machines and programs will serve to unlock the hidden potential in severely disabled students. That's good news, because it means that as many as 50 different manufacturers and some 500 software producers can be used as sources of classroom materials.

Sometimes, though, specialized devices are needed. This happened, for example, at the Easter Seals school in Little Rock, Arkansas. Bob Taylor, who is responsible for the school's computer-related functions, is becoming very frustrated as he sees how limited some of the available equipment is when used in special education. Taylor and a team of classroom teachers and therapists work with severely disabled children whose handicaps range from cerebral palsy to retardation.

I watched as 12 year-old Carrie had a "speech therapy" session. It was a painful experience. Carrie, who has cerebral palsy, communicated with her therapist, Rachel, by hitting her head on a securely mounted lever switch placed on the lapboard of her wheelchair. Each bang of the head produced a different light signal. Rachel knew what each signal meant. Rachel then placed a Zygo Industries E-tran™ communicator on Carrie's lapboard. The E-tran is a transparent stand-up screen with one- and two-word messages handwritten at different points on the screen. In response to Rachel's questions, Carrie would look at first one message and then another; Rachel could see the identical messages on her side of the screen.

Both communication systems required a skilled therapist, such as Rachel, who knew Carrie very well and who posed specific questions so as to frame a context in which to interpret the child's short responses. Even so, Rachel often has to guess what Carrie is trying to say. And Carrie seldom can use these systems except with family members, teachers, or close friends.

Taylor then took me to a different room, where I met 13-year-old

Chris, a bright, alert boy who has cerebral palsy. Taylor explained that Chris had learned to use an Apple computer by moving a small magnet over the top of a special interface (go-between) device called an Autocom. The $6,000 Autocom, marketed by Prentke Romich, and a similar machine, the Tetrascan™ sold by Zygo Industries, contain keyboard "emulators." As illustrated in Figure 4.1, the combination of devices, in this case the Tetrascan working with a Franklin Ace 1000 computer, allows someone like Chris to compose a message of his own by selecting words on the emulator, which then transmits the text to the computer.

Chris was watching us, understanding everything we were saying. I walked over to his chair. "How do you like the Autocom, Chris?" I asked. His eyes gleaming, he turned immediately to his lapboard, on which was displayed an array of words, letters, and numbers. Moving his hand slowly, he took almost three minutes to answer me: "I think it takes two percent as long as a typewriter." The clarity and precision of his reply made me intensely conscious of the difference between Chris's intellectual functioning and his ability to communicate quickly.

Until you see children such as Chris and Carrie, you may not realize how much of a "hands on" experience education really is. We learn, not just by listening to teachers and reading books, but by doing things with our hands, bodies, and objects in our environments. We interact with our world and thereby master it. Chris and Carrie have the intelligence, hearing, and vision they need to engage in productive education in the passive sense. What's holding them back is their inability to manipulate objects, numbers, and words quickly and easily in a creative manner.

The gift of the microcomputer in special education for such children is its capacity to facilitate creative learning. As long as Carrie is restricted to noncomputer communication technologies, she faces barriers in the simplest tasks. Suppose you were Carrie. You'd be able to request a drink, indicate that you wished to visit the restroom, convey the desire to take a rest, and answer questions with "Yes," "No," or similar one- and two-word responses. You'd be able to do this only with a few people. And you'd have to endure, even with these close friends, endless misinterpretations of your meaning until they finally understood what you wanted to say.

Or think of Nancy Sopp's students, unable to read grade-level books and manuals. They may be in junior high school, but, without some means of interacting more easily and directly with information, they will not be able to work at the junior high school level.

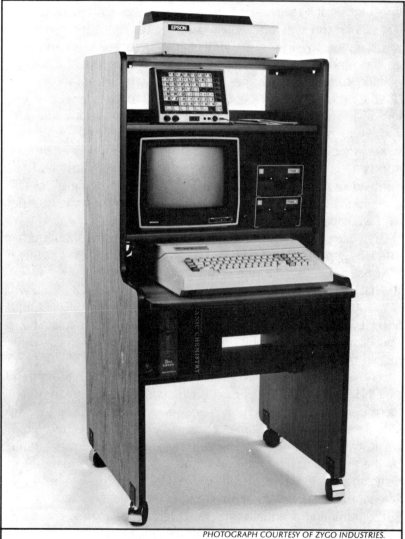

PHOTOGRAPH COURTESY OF ZYGO INDUSTRIES.

Figure 4.1: *The Tetrascan^TM by Zygo Industries, shown with a Franklin Ace 1000, a monitor, two disk drives, and a printer.*

The need for creative and expressive ways to communicate is an important reason for the popularity of the LOGO computer language with learning-disabled children and youth. Reports James Muller, a Richardson, Texas, father of a learning-disabled 16-year-old son: "I became fascinated with Larry's approach to the computer. He saw it for what it really is—a tool. And that is exactly how he used it."

Muller's son was once diagnosed as retarded. It's a common mistake, one physicians frequently make, because both learning disabilities and general retardation produce symptoms of a seeming inability to learn, lack of interest in the environment, and the like. But the two are very different. In learning disabilities, a specific intellectual function is disrupted; usually, as in dyslexia, it is the serial processing of words that is impaired. At other times the processing of sounds or other symbols may be dysfunctional. Retardation, by contrast, is a general limitation in functioning. Most learning-disabled persons display normal intelligence in doing all but the affected activities, while retarded individuals demonstrate less-than-average capabilities across a range of functions.

That Larry is not retarded is evident today. A high school student, he earns good grades. And one reason, his father believes, is that he now has a tool that lets him create.

That tool is a personal computer equipped with LOGO. And what is LOGO? It is a programming language, much as BASIC, COBOL, and PILOT are languages. LOGO uses a "turtle" (a triangular-shaped "pen") to produce graphic images on a computer screen. Unlike most other computer programming languages, LOGO uses few letters and words. BASIC, for example, uses such commands as LIN$(J+D)=T$. A dyslexic child would have problems with these commands, although, as Nancy Sopp demonstrates, the child would eventually learn some of them. LOGO bypasses the difficult BASIC-type commands to allow a child to create with images formed by the "turtle," which the child moves around the screen. As the turtle moves, it leaves a trail. By manipulating the shape on the screen, the child creates an image.

Programming is equally simple. LOGO's commands use only a few words. TO SQUARE, for example, might be used. The child would tell the computer to move the turtle forward ten spaces by typing FD 10. To have the turtle to make a right turn at a 90-degree angle, all that is necessary is to type RT 90. A few more commands telling the computer to move the turtle forward and to turn right two more times completes the program. Then, when the child wishes to produce a square, he merely types SQUARE and hits ENTER. The computer does the rest.

Is this merely glorified drawing? To the child, it probably is. But the teacher knows that the exercise is tapping skills in arithmetic, geometry, and, yes, English. Perhaps most important, the child is creating in a way as easy for him as writing a short story might be for another child. LOGO commands are executed as soon as the child presses ENTER. It's that easy—and fast. For children with short attention spans or low frustration tolerances, such quick and competent reactions produce intense satisfaction. The child is succeeding at doing something by himself; for many disabled children, that is a rare experience. They are doing things that are, in psychological jargon, positively reinforced. For children using LOGO, they are also doing more of something their parents and teachers greatly value: they are learning.

In Pennsylvania, Eldred Township Elementary School teacher Margaret Smith knows the value of pride in achievement. Last year, she won a statewide competition for a grant enabling her to purchase a microcomputer and printer to use with her 38 mentally retarded and learning disabled students. "We had only $250 to order supplies this year," she says, referring to Eldred Township's budget for school equipment. That's why the $3,700 award was so important. She competed with 2,500 other teachers to get one of the 253 awards granted by the state education department. Mrs. Smith believes the computer has already made a difference for her students: "A computer can be programmed to make positive responses, no matter how many mistakes the student makes." And her students have something special to show off: "They can say, 'Look, we have a computer and the other students don't.' Let's face it: there's not a whole lot our kids can do that others can't."

Sue Prince, a speech pathologist working with retarded children at the Cerebral Palsy Center in Belleville, New Jersey, adds: "Large amounts of time and patience, which we can't always provide, are required for some students to learn even basic concepts. But the computer will sit there very patiently going over and over those concepts."

The microcomputer can do something else that is vital to education: it can help expand a child's horizons. Special education literature is filled with references to "experiential deprivation" in handicapped children and youth. The forbidding term merely means that the children have not had the same range of opportunities to explore the world as have other children their age. But with a computer, even severely disabled children can experience things they need to learn about.

Computer simulation is being used today to train airline pilots. Before the pilot steps into the cockpit of a 767, for example, he or she has spent hundreds of hours in front of a simulator that presents for study and immediate reaction a whole range of possible problems and disasters. As a result, the new pilot has already "been there" when, for example, an electrical storm interferes with navigation. For the deaf students at Mill Neck Manor School on Long Island, New York, the microcomputer plays a similar role. By using school-written programs such as Our Town and Supermarket Craze, says curriculum director Lou Frillman, students can learn how to locate the community services they need. When they go to local stores on supervised excursions, they're already familiar with the area.

But perhaps the most dramatic use of microcomputers in special education is to do what handicapped children are unable to do by themselves. Today's personal computers can be adapted to read for blind students, write for paralyzed or mobility-limited students, speak for children unable to talk, and, at least to some extent, hear for deaf students. Let's look for a moment at some of these capabilities.

Speech Synthesis

How can a computer "talk"?

People who use speech sythesizers are so accustomed to hearing artificial speech (as when a Chrysler enunciates "Fasten seat belt" or "Thank you") that they seldom stop to think about how the computer accomplishes this task. The ways in which it is done become important because the technologies carry with them, together with remarkable promise, some unexpected pitfalls.

The Echo II and Votrax Type-'N-Talk™ speech synthesizers are quite inexpensive, both selling for under $250. They represent the "low end" of the market. I asked Larry Skutchan, a graduate student at the University of Arkansas at Little Rock, to demonstrate the Echo II for me in his trailer home. As Larry started typing, I watched my interpreter to see how clear the speech was. One look at the consternation on her face was enough to give me my answer. Larry laughed. "It takes a while, Frank. I spent ten hours at the machine before the speech became easily comprehensible." I asked him if the Votrax sounded like the Echo. "Yeah, it's about the same. With speech synthesizers, you get what you pay for. The more expensive units sound a lot better."

There are basically three ways a computer talks.

Votrax's Type-'N-Talk, illustrated in Figure 4.2, uses what is called "phoneme coding." The system stores basic speech sounds and rules for stringing them together into words. The sounds and rules are stored in computer memory chips. Type-'N-Talk uses only a little of the computer's memory to produce an almost unlimited number of sound combinations. For all intents and purposes, then, the Votrax's vocabulary is unlimited.

Why not store complete words, properly pronounced? The answer is simple. To do so would take up so much of the computer's memory that it would not be possible to run any programs on the machine.

The Type-'N-Talk unit is produced by Votrax, a division in the Michigan-based Federal Screw Works. For more information, write Votrax Consumer Products Group (500 Stephenson Highway, Troy, MI 48084).

The Echo II speech synthesizer uses technology developed by Texas Instruments (TI) called "linear predictive coding." The TI chip stores an electronic model of the human vocal tract together with digital versions of pitch and energy level. A text-to-speech software program contains hundreds of language and pronunciation rules; for this reason, there is no fixed vocabulary. The phonemes generated by the text-to-speech program are converted to sound by the TI chip, and the sound is amplified by a speaker. The Echo II is priced below the Type-'N-Talk, retailing for under $200. For more information, contact Street Electronics Corporation (1140 Mark Ave., Carpenteria, CA 93013).

A third technology, National Semiconductor's "wave-form digitization," produces good quality speech but uses a lot of computer memory to do so. The pitch, or frequency, of speech is broken down into digital pulses (computers can read only digital messages, basically a series of "0" and "1" strings) and stored. When text is read, the pulses are brought together again to form words. Because the system uses considerable computer memory (more than most 8-bit machines have available), and because of the high cost of the technology (as much as $4,000), this approach is one not often used in education.

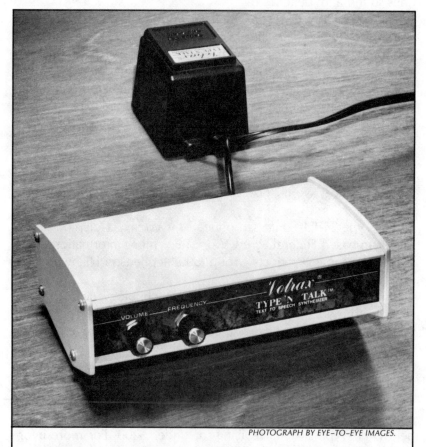

PHOTOGRAPH BY EYE–TO–EYE IMAGES.

Figure 4.2: *Votrax Type-'N-Talk™, a speech synthesizer.*

Three limitations characterize the speech-synthesizer technologies. First, the systems use software. This means they are not compatible with protected software, such as Wordstar or Visicalc. They may be used with user-written software or with unprotected software. They may also be used with software specifically written to be run with speech synthesizers.

A second limitation is characteristic of the industry as a whole: hardware and software are often incompatible. So it is with some speech synthesizers. The Echo II, for example, will work only with Apple computers; if you have an IBM, you can use the Echo PC, or if you have some other microcomputer, the Echo GP may be what you want.

The third major limitation relates to the first. Whether user-developed or specially written for use with a synthesizer, software must restrict itself to readable information. No speech synthesizer available today, to my knowledge, can read computer graphics or other images. Were the students to try, the speech synthesizer simply would read each character and each line one by one.

The industry is responding to the problems and limitations associated with speech-output technology in some interesting ways. The need for high-quality speech conflicts, as I have shown, with the memory requirements of much educational and other software. At Borg Warner Educational Systems, an elegant solution has been found to this problem, at least with respect to Apple II and IIe computers. The company's Ufonic™ Voice System has its own self-contained memory. The interface card containing the synthesizer also has a microprocessor and sufficient memory to run the synthesizer; it is, in effect, a computer within a computer. By using its own memory, the Ufonic system can generate good speech without robbing the computer of the memory it needs to run complex educational programs.

Eydie Sloane, a computer-training specialist with the Dade County, Florida, public schools, reports that the Ufonic system produces speech much clearer than that available with most other system. Says Sloane, a natural enthusiast: "I'm wildly impressed with the Ufonic voice programs from Borg Warner. They came out with a product I think is super. Definitely look for it. About $500, but what a great sound! No mechanical voice. Just nice and easy, good quality and in English or Spanish (in Miami, that's a real necessity)." For more information about Ufonic, contact Borg Warner Educational Systems (600 W. University Drive, Arlington Heights, IL 60004).

Late in 1983 Digital Equipment Corporation (DEC) announced another intriguing approach to the problems characterizing synthesized speech. DECtalk™, a $4,000 unit, will plug into virtually any computer. And the speech quality is excellent; so good is it, in fact, that MCI Communications Corporation is using it with its MCI Mail electronic mail service. The DEC system adds inflections to speech and can vary its speed from 120 to 350 words per minute. For blind persons who need to do a great deal of reading of computer-stored information, the combination of clarity and speed is a godsend. Conversational speech usually runs at about 180 words per minute, but psychological research has established that the brain can absorb and interpret information spoken much faster than that; in fact, one reason some students become bored in class is that their minds are left free to roam in irrelevant (to the teacher!) ways during a typical lecture. At 300 words per minute, though, near-total attention is required. Blind individuals who have made their way through law school, with its voluminous reading requirements, tell me that their use of tape recorders with double-conversational-speed playback capabilities increased their retention of information and saved enormous amounts of time. At $4,000, however, DECtalk is more likely to be used in resource rooms at schools and universities than at home.

Both DECtalk and Ufonic have speech quality sufficiently good for another educational purpose: giving voice to nonvocal students. Carrie and Chris at the Little Rock, Arkansas, Easter Seals school, for instance, could use such technologies to communicate with persons unskilled in interpreting their speech. They could, for example, compose a message on a computer (using a special device like the Autocom) and send it via telephone to others, without the need to ask a teacher or parent to make the call for them. Boston's Children's Hospital uses DECtalk with speech-impaired children; when the children touch the screen, the computer says the word being touched.

Educators may find, too, as Dr. Sloane does in Miami, that such high-quality speech synthesizers can be used to add voice to teacher-written instructional programs. Such talking software would be a boon for dyslexic and blind students.

Maryland Computer Services is taking a third approach to the problems of the speech synthesizers. The company markets a complete system consisting of a Hewlett-Packard 125 computer especially equipped with high-quality speech capabilities. The model, called Information Through Speech™ (ITS), shown in Figure 4.3, can read punctuation, upper- and lower-case letters, and numbers; it can read words as units or spell them out. Speed is controlled by the user and can range as high as 700 words per minute. The machine runs popular programs with no incompatibility problems due to the speech-synthesis unit; this opens the way to the use of thousands of pieces of software. Also available from the company is its own software, for example, a form writer. Prices for the ITS range from about $8,000 to about $12,000; the latter price includes a hard disk drive capability.

In Butler, New Jersey, the National Institute for Rehabilitation Engineering (NIRE) makes available a specially modified TRS-80 Radio

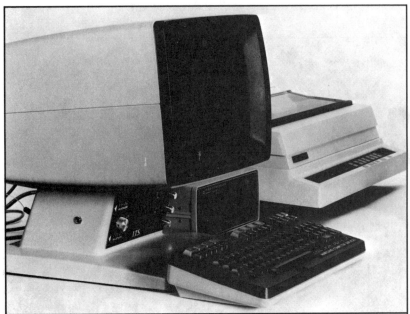

PHOTOGRAPH © 1982 TADDER/BALTIMORE, COURTESY OF MARYLAND COMPUTER SERVICES, INC.

Figure 4.3: Information Through Speech™ (ITS), a talking computer marketed by Maryland Computer Services, with a printer.

Shack Model III that NIRE calls the "Talking Typewriter." In addition to speech synthesis, the machine displays words and numbers in extra-large type for the benefit of people who have some usable vision. NIRE's version of the Model III also requires two-key, rather than one-key, operation of the ESC (escape) and BREAK keys, so that blind users will not lose material by striking these keys by mistake. The system, including the Model III, a printer, and a cassette drive (a disk drive also is available), costs $1,895. For more information, contact NIRE (97 Decker Rd., Butler, NJ 07405).

The work of Indiana's Bill Grimm, shown in Figure 4.4, represents another approach to the problems facing speech-synthesizer users. Grimm, founder of Computer Aids Corporation, is something of a legend among blind computer users. Of the several dozen blind individuals using Apple computers and Echo II speech synthesizers I talked with while preparing this book, all but one mentioned Grimm. Bob Taylor, the Easter Seals educator in Little Rock, explains the basic reason: "At least, Grimm's got the software." What Grimm has done is to assemble a package of an Apple II computer

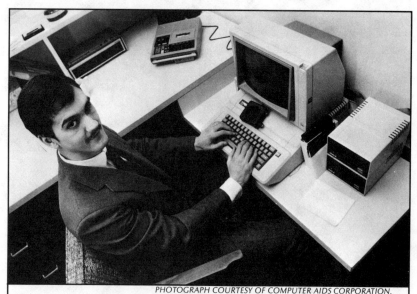

PHOTOGRAPH COURTESY OF COMPUTER AIDS CORPORATION.

Figure 4.4: Computer Aids head Bill Grimm, shown using an Apple computer, the Echo II speech synthesizer, and a tape recorder.

(usually the IIe), an Echo II, and his own word-processing and other software programs specifically written for use with both pieces of hardware. He also has software that enables blind persons using the Echo II to tap into The Source and CompuServe, two popular database and bulletin-board services: such services broaden the "library" available to a child several thousandfold, because these services (with the Echo II and Grimm's programs) let blind and dyslexic individuals "read" the *New York Times*, the Associated Press or United Press International wire sevices, and the information stored on dozens of computerized data bases. Contact Grimm at Computer Aids (4929 South Lafayette St., Fort Wayne, IN 46806).

Is it possible to link the inexpensive Votrax or Echo II speech synthesizer technology to "protected" software? By doing so, we would be helping many individuals obtain an affordable at-home system they could use for schoolwork. The need for such a development is obvious. First, the high-quality speech systems, such as those marketed by Maryland Computer Services, DEC, and others, while good, are probably too expensive for many families to purchase. And second, schools are increasingly using protected software programs in the classroom—and expecting students to use them at home as well. Locking blind and dyslexic students out of this rich lode of programs defeats the concept of integration in education that is at the heart of today's special education programming.

One person who recognizes the need and is doing something about it is University of Illinois law professor Peter Maggs. I asked Maggs to explain the issues involved: "The software for the Echo II and for systems using the Votrax rely upon the Apple or other computer's operating system functioning in its normal manner. 'Protected software' often alters or disables the operating system so that the user cannot use the operating system to copy the software." What's he doing about it? "I am now looking into possibilities of providing a hardware solution to this problem. The hardware solution would physically intercept signals from the keyboard to the screen and so would not have to interface directly with the operating system." It is an ingenious approach. Maggs' work, conducted with his colleagues at Visek and Maggs, a small company that has done considerable work on speech technology for major computer companies, received funds from the U.S. Department of Education to develop a prototype speech-synthesis chip that one of the dozen synthesizer manufacturers could produce in quantity at a manufacturing cost of under $50. Maggs hopes to provide units that will work with the IBM PC, the Apple IIe, and the TRS-80 Model 100 computers.

A different set of issues emerges when speech synthesizer technologies are applied to meet the special education needs of retarded students.

Before getting into these problems, I need to make the point that educable mentally retarded children and youth can use personal computers—and use them well. This is evident to many parents, but, because of the "high tech" image of computers, you might not expect that such sophisticated devices could be used independently by persons with severe retardation. However, not only can retarded persons use computers, but mounting evidence indicates that many retarded students learn better with computers than with almost any other educational technology. This is primarily because of the computer's "patience," but also because of the interactive nature of good computer instruction, the rapid feedback to the user, and the applicability of interesting sights and sounds to reach the student's mind.

Research conducted by the late Marc Gold, an expert on teaching retarded individuals, demonstrates that when information is broken down into small units and each unit is taught separately, retarded individuals can learn things previously thought to be beyond their ken. This knowledge is now being tapped to use microcomputers as tools for teaching retarded children and youth. At Indianhead Enterprises, a center for developmentally disabled students in Menomonie, Wisconsin, Sam Jenkins and his colleagues conducted a study to see if severely retarded students, whose measured I.Q.'s ranged from 30 to 88, could be taught the location and use of the keys on a computer keyboard. A Texas Instruments 99/4A home computer displayed an image of the keyboard on its screen, randomly flashing individual keys on and off. A synthesized voice told the student which key to press. Meanwhile, the computer automatically tallied the right/wrong responses and with the speech synthesizer told the student the results: "Right!" or "No, try again." Jenkins and his team found, perhaps surprisingly, that performance by the students was not related in any statistically significant way to their I.Q.'s. Most students, though, did learn the location of most keys, even in the five-minute test period. Speech synthesis and nonverbal cues appear particularly well suited to helping retarded children, many of whom have extremely limited reading abilities.

Jenkins' favorable experiences with retarded and learning-disabled students led him to form a small company designed to develop educational materials for these populations. One such program, called Keyboard Trainer, teaches children to use the computer keyboard by telling them, via the synthesizer, what each key does and where it is located. Early Counting Fun and Fish and Count, two counting programs, also use the synthesizer. Jenkins sells the programs at prices ranging from $15 to $30. For more information, contact The Upper Room (907 6th Avenue East, Menomonie, WI 54751).

Speech Recognition

A "sister technology" to speech synthesis is voice or speech recognition. How does a computer "hear"? So far, not very well. But important progress is being made. Speech recognition is of most use now to physically disabled students who are not able to manipulate the keyboard with authority. It is also helpful as a relatively easy way to get the computer to perform certain functions, regardless of the user's disability. Computers today are capable of recognizing and responding to a few hundred words, usually words spoken by a single person.

Speech recognition is accomplished by microcomputers in several fairly complicated fashions. Most popular by far, at this early stage in development, is the technology that creates a "template" (computer-readable version) of individual words. Each template essentially is a sequence of numbers; remember, computers can only read bits (series of "0" and "1" numerals). The user speaks the words, one by one, into a microphone or other input mechanism; some systems require that each word be entered several times. The computer then translates these sounds into number-based templates and stores them. Later, when the user is running a program and enunciates a word, the computer searches among all its templates to find one that matches what it has just heard. That word will be displayed and, if appropriate, the command will be executed. What happens if the person speaks a word not recognized by the computer? The answer is a simple one: nothing.

The template-based speech recognition systems can handle only a few words because storing each one requires an enormous amount of computer memory. The speech-recognition system that Texas Instruments recently announced for use with its Professional Computer samples speech sounds an astounding 8,000 times per second in order to construct a reliable template. Says Robert Schadewald, who has studied speech-recognition technologies: "Trying to apply methods that work for limited vocabularies to average speaking vocabularies of 3,000 to 8,000 words may be like trying to build a long-bow with a 50-mile range." Clearly, template-based technologies are limited to small vocabularies.

A different approach, being researched at Carnegie-Mellon University, is called "feature extraction." In this system, the computer attempts to recognize the numerical patterns of sound and to use these to identify the individual words being used. And what are these patterns? Anyone who recalls seeing spectrograms knows that speech can be displayed in two dimensions, those of frequency (pitch) and time. What a feature extractor does, in effect, is to compare the spectrogram (reduced to numbers, of course) of a word to a number sequence in its memory. If it finds a match, it displays the word (by sending a digital version of the word to a dictionary, which converts the digits into an English word). If appropriate, the computer also executes the command.

Speech recognition now is being used in a number of interesting ways. For example, AT&T Bell Laboratories got into the business of speech-recognition research for a simple reason. The company wanted telephone users to be able to speak commands to a phone, have it understand the instructions, search its memory, and automatically dial the call. Two sets of research studies were conducted for many years before yielding results: one explored number recognition while the other examined letter recognition. AT&T expects that by 1986, if not earlier, affordable units will be on the market that will allow a user to speak either the telephone number or the called party's name; the phone would do the rest. The company's products will likely be speaker-dependent, which means that the telephone will recognize only one voice; speaker-independent versions also are planned but probably will recognize fewer words. Just two weeks after AT&T's pending products were revealed, ITT announced a speaker-independent telephone, also slated for the market within a few years. And then, in early summer 1984, small Entrex Electronics introduced a $325 telephone that understands a few words. The machine, first announced in March and expected to be in stores by the time you read this, responds first to the word "Phone." In effect, saying "Phone" while standing in the room gets the device's attention. If you then say "Mom," for example, it will automatically search its memory for your mother's telephone number and then dial that number. For more information, contact Entrex Electronics (839 S. Beacon St., San Pedro, CA 90731). What this development means for severely physically disabled individuals who have difficulty moving quickly is that they can initiate and answer telephone calls without even touching the phone.

At Scott Instruments, a Texas company specializing in speech-recognition products, a fairly inexpensive ($595) system capable of handling as many as 1,000 words per disk, Shadow/VET™, is now available. Used with an Apple II Plus computer, the system makes the Apple "think" that the information is being put into the computer by means of the keyboard. The Shadow/VET terminal (VET stands for "voice entry terminal") holds up to 40 words in memory at any given time; a simple command calls up additional 40-word vocabularies, as many as 25 on each disk, as needed.

To understand how important something like the Shadow/VET terminal can be for a physically disabled student, consider the use of The Source, the popular information data bank. To call up The Source using the keyboard requires as many as 80 different keystrokes; for someone with severe arthritis or other physical disability, that would be difficult, if not impossible. Using the Shadow/VET terminal, however, requires just four spoken commands: "Source," "log on," "sign on," and then the function such as "UPI" to get the United Press International wire service data.

As I noted earlier, high-quality speech-synthesis systems require a lot of memory. Wouldn't something like the Shadow/VET terminal also need a great deal of memory? Yes, of course. But Scott Instruments has taken the approach Borg Warner adopted for the Ufonic synthesizer: Scott placed the 16K memory that the Shadow/VET system needs on its own board, so the Apple doesn't need to lend any of its memory for the digital signal and recognition capabilities. For more information, contact Scott Instruments (1111 Willow Springs Drive, Denton, TX 76205).

To date, it has been particularly difficult to do spreadsheet analysis by voice. Now, Supersoft Inc. offers ScratchPad with VoiceDrive™, a product designed to provide an interface, or go-between, that works with the spreadsheet software program and the voice-recognition module. The $495 program is compatible with Tecmar's PC-Mate Voice Recognition Board™ and with Texas Instruments' Speech Command System. Supersoft offers a complete package of PC-Mate and ScratchPad with VoiceDrive for $995. For more information, contact Supersoft (PO Box 1628, Champaign, IL 61820).

The Texas Instruments speech-recognition board is actually two cards placed on one slot within the Professional Computer. One card handles the sending and receiving of the signal; the other takes care of processing the information. The linear predictive-coding pattern used to recognize words may also be used to regenerate the speech signal itself. The quality of the system, which add some $3,000 to the Professional Computer's price, is excellent. Says Robb Aley Allan, who reviewed the computer for *Popular Computing's* October 1983 issue: "The reproduction is like that of a good connection on a long-distance telephone call." For more information, contact Texas Instruments (P.O. Box 402430, Dallas, TX 75240).

Interstate Electronics, a unit of Figgie International, markets speech-recognition chips primarily to original equipment manufacturers (OEMs) rather than to retail customers. If you are sophisticated about the workings of your personal computer, however, you might want to contact the company about its products (Interstate Electronics Corporation, P.O. Box 3117, Anaheim, CA 92803).

A number of speech-recognition programs are marketed specifically for use in education. One of these is Scott Instruments' Voice Based Learning System™ (VBLS), which is designed for teachers and parents who wish to write their own instructional programs. Retailing at $100, VBLS can be used with the Shadow/VET to add voice to teacher-written software. The instructional packages would recognize and respond to what the student is able to generate. Say, for example, that a cerebral palsy student typically says "staw" for "stop." The program can be set to respond to "staw"; if, however, the objective is to train the person to speak more clearly, the teacher, therapist, or parent can set the system to respond only to the version of the word that represents the student's best pronunciation.

John Williams would have found such a system ideal for his purposes. Williams, who lives in Sterling, Virginia, has spent enough money over the past three decades for speech therapy to enable him to purchase a hundred VBLS systems. With typical good humor, though, Williams accepts my suggestion that he use the program for self-therapy to control his stuttering. Right now, Williams uses an Epson QX-10™ computer for his extensive freelance writing, fund raising, and consultation duties as head of Technical Communications, Inc., the Virginia-based communications company that publishes the monthly *Special Needs Computing*. The VBLS would not work with an Epson, but it would work with an Apple or an Apple-compatible machine, such as the Franklin 1000. Is he willing to convert? "I'll give it a try, Frank. I've stuttered all my life. I have never enjoyed it. I have damned it, detested it, slept with it, carried it like a shield for everyone to see, been ridiculed for it more times than I want to remember. One thing is for sure. My wife will appreciate my practicing on a machine so she doesn't have to listen to all my starts and stops."

Williams is one of the most determined people I know—and his wife Lisa one of the most patient. Their experiences illustrate something few people understand about speech-related disabilities: speech is a motor activity. As such, it involves fine coordination of an entire phalanx of muscles. Those muscles respond to only one thing: habit. Most are not even under voluntary control. Despite his intelligence, John still has difficulty controlling his stuttering even after a successful career in public relations and journalism. The personal computer can help John by responding only to correctly pronounced words and phrases. If he uses the system enough, he will be forced to speak clearly if he wants to get anything done. By tying his speech quality directly to his work output, the program would reinforce John for good speech while disregarding, in a nonjudgmental way, his mistakes.

Because John does so much writing, I suggested he look, as well, at Serota Engineering's C2E2 system. Designed for use by physically disabled individuals, the $400 package features what Serota calls Textwriter, a program that handles word processing entirely by voice. Textwriter combines a modification of a commercial word-processing program with the Shadow/VET system, available as an extra-cost option from Serota or from Scott. A severely disabled individual unable to use a keyboard would be able to write class assignments, notes, and other materials entirely by speaking, although frequent changing of the limited vocabulary recognized by the Shadow/VET would be required. C2E2 (Communications, environmental Control, Education, and Entertainment) is available from Serota Engineering Consultants (3730 Alta Crest Drive, P.O. Box 43286, Birmingham, AL 35243).

MCE, Inc. and The Conover Company both distribute Voice Machine Communications' Voice Input Module™ (VIM), which works with Apple II-type computers, including the Franklin 1000. VIM is shown in Figures 4.5 and 4.6. What makes the under-$1,000 VIM interesting is that an unlimited number of 80-word subsets may be used, giving the operator a virtually unlimited vocabulary. Like other commerically available speech-recognition systems, VIM

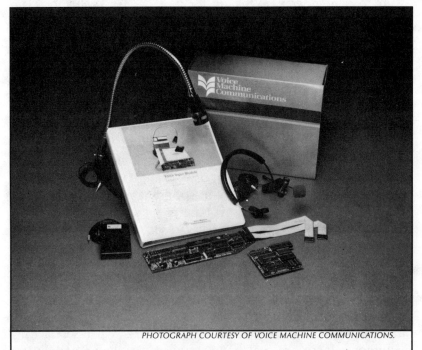

PHOTOGRAPH COURTESY OF VOICE MACHINE COMMUNICATIONS.

Figure 4.5: Voice Machine Communications' Voice Input Module for the Intro Voice System™.

recognizes only the user who trains it. Duane Phillips of MCE claims that the VIM can perform at more than a 98 percent level of accuracy in recognizing words. He notes that, for students unable to use a keyboard, speech-limited individuals, and others, VIM offers the ability to bypass complex keyboard-entry commands: "Since voice input virtually eliminates the need to learn specific keyboard commands, students may be introduced at an earlier age or at a more conceptual level to such complex software applications as computer-aided design (CAD), database and word processing." For more information, contact Voice Machine Communications (1000 S. Grand, Santa Ana, CA 92705); MCE, Inc. (157 S. Kalamazoo Mall, Kalamazoo, MI 49007); or The Conover Company (P.O. Box 155, Omro, WI 54963).

Such products as VIM and Shadow/VET presumably could also be used by dyslexic and retarded individuals to control computer

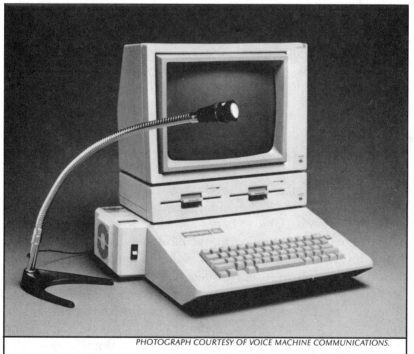

PHOTOGRAPH COURTESY OF VOICE MACHINE COMMUNICATIONS.

Figure 4.6: The Intro Voice System^{TM} with an Apple computer.

programs. These students often find it much more difficult to use words and letters in writing than to speak them. Sam Jenkins of The Upper Room is one person who might be contacted for information about such applications.

But what about deaf students? Ultimately, the ability of the computer to "hear" is going to revolutionize education, and just about everything else, for deaf persons. But that day is at least five to ten years away.

As we have seen, most commercially available systems are speaker-dependent. The cost seems out of line for an application in which the deaf person would use VIM or Shadow/VET to understand just one other individual. Speaker-independent systems remain limited in vocabulary, making their application to education for deaf students of little value. However, to the extent that a program such as Scott Instruments' VBLS is used to help deaf students learn to speak more clearly, speech recognition already has a place in education for deaf children.

This is not to imply that the role of personal computers in the education of deaf students is restricted; in fact, quite the opposite is true. Of all severely handicapped people, deaf individuals are probably the most likely to benefit from computer-aided instruction. However, for the next few years at least, speech recognition will not be one of the reasons deaf students take so well to microcomputers.

Keyboard Emulators

As we have seen, many severely disabled children have difficulty manipulating the standard computer keyboard. For these students, "emulators" are available to offer alternative ways of entering information into, and controlling the action of, a computer. The term simply means that the device makes the computer "think" that its own keyboard is being used; in effect, the peripheral product "emulates" the keyboard.

Speech-input systems, such as VIM, contain emulators. So, too, can joysticks, familiar to most readers as the means by which many computer games are played, be used with emulators. Severely disabled persons may also use the Autocom, as does Little Rock's Chris, to operate an Apple or similar computer; the $6,000 device is distributed by Prentke Romich, a company that is prominent in any discussion of keyboard emulators. It is also available from The Trace R&D Center at the University of Wisconsin–Madison, a major center of activity in the area of emulators.

What is the Autocom? It is a large, magnet-sensitive electronic board for communication by nonvocal individuals. The Autocom has its own screen, across which words and phrases scroll much as they do on a computer screen, except that the Autocom displays large characters and only one line at a time. Cerebral palsy, quadriplegia, severe arthritis, and other fine-motor-control related disabilities often interfere with computer-keyboard operation, but, with the Autocom, all that is required is to grasp a magnet about the size of a joint on your finger and move it onto the square containing the word, number, or phrase one wishes to communicate. As Chris in Little Rock showed us, the Autocom can be used with a keyboard emulator by individuals who lack the manual dexterity to manipulate a keyboard.

Why does such a fairly simple communicator cost twice as much as a fully equipped Apple II? The reason goes back to the nature of "special" equipment. Only a few Autocoms are sold each year, which means that the entire cost of development, manufacturing, marketing, and distribution must be spread across a few units of sales. Fortunately, Prentke Romich, which distributes the communicator, provides excellent after-purchase support through approved vendors.

The Autocom is an example of a "direct-select" aid that will drive a keyboard emulator. The individual points directly to the letter, number, word, or phrase desired. Whenever it is possible, such a mechanism should be used. Both Prentke Romich and Trace R&D Center distribute a rather dazzling range of pointer technologies that are usable with direct-select emulators: a joystick, a light pen, a mouthstick, a tongue switch, and a pneumatic puff-and-sip switch. Figure 4.7 shows Mike Ward using a light pen. Which switch or set of switches is used depends on the user's limitations. Severely impaired children can use tongue or puff-and-sip controls if they have little or no upper-limb mobility; less disabled students can manipulate joysticks or the Autocom's magnet by hand.

Some children, however, are so severely disabled that they cannot easily use direct-select technologies. Gregg Vanderheiden, director of the Trace Center, and others have devised ingenious two-step

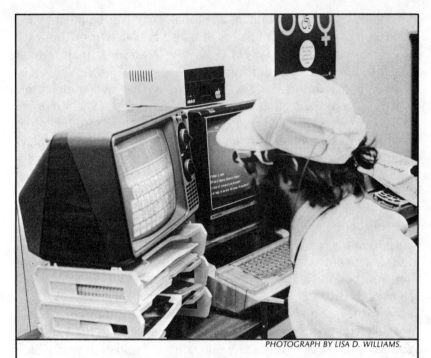

PHOTOGRAPH BY LISA D. WILLIAMS.

Figure 4.7: Mike Ward uses a light pen attached to his hat to run a "menu" program. When the light remains on a letter or number for five seconds, the character is entered into the progam.

or even multi-step scanning technologies these children can use. Such approaches often use menu-driven software. The child needs to select the first letter of a word or string of words. Immediately following that selection, the screen displays a set of pre-entered words beginning with that letter. In some programs, these words (or phrases, if desired) are numbered, and the child selects the appropriate number.

With so many different hardware and software approaches available from some two dozen vendors, teachers and parents are well advised to ask such experts as Prentke Romich's Barry Romich or Trace's Gregg Vanderheiden to assemble a system for a particular child. Contact Prentke Romich (8769 Township Rd. 513, Shreve, OH 44676-9421) or Trace R&D Center (University of Wisconsin–Madison, 314 Waisman Center, 1500 Highland Ave., Madison, WI 53706). Also available from Trace is an "International Software/Hardware

Directory," a loose-leaf binder collection of brief descriptions of different approaches.

Gregg Vanderheiden is interested in finding ways to speed up computer input by severely disabled, nonvocal children and adults. As we saw in Little Rock with Chris, pointing to individual letters and words consumes an inordinate amount of time. But there is another problem that Vanderheiden is now tackling, with support from the U.S. Department of Education. To illustrate the problem, and Vanderheiden's approach, imagine for a moment that you are Chris in Little Rock. In our hypothetical illustration, you are writing a report using the Autocom as your keyboard emulator with the Apple computer. Suppose you need to calculate some numbers to put into the report. Can you use your personal computer to do that? Yes, but it would take time. First, you'd have to give the word-processing program some "end session" commands and remove the disk from the computer. Then you would insert another disk, this one having a program that runs calculations. After doing the arithmetic, you'd remove that disk and substitute your original word-processing disk on the computer. All of this takes a great deal of time—and you've lost your place in the word-processing program.

This is a serious matter for many thousands of children with cerebral palsy and other severe disabilities that interfere with speech. It is particularly troublesome because the personal computer is used to perform so many basic functions for these children in the classroom; the students use it not only to do schoolwork, but also to communicate with others in the room.

Fortunately, this problem is rapidly being solved by some of the newer personal computers. With Apple's new Macintosh, for example, you can interrupt a word-processing program, "mark your place," shift to a calculation or graphics program, complete that task, and then bring the results of your work (the numbers or the images) into the report you are writing. This capability is, of course, useful for people who are not disabled. For severely impaired individuals, however, it is more than useful: it comes close to being essential.

Keyboard Modifications

For some disabled children, modifications in the computer itself may be preferable to the use of an emulator. The most obvious example is to place a keyguard over the keyboard. IBM, for example, makes keyguards for its Selectric typewriters and sells them for about $10 each. The plastic boards contain holes over the keys; striking the wrong key becomes much more difficult. With computer keyboards, a second issue emerges. Some of the most commonly used commands require that two keys be pressed at once. With an Apple, for example, you can make the cursor (the small, flashing light that tells you where you are on the screen) move in one direction by pressing CONTROL and A simultaneously. Many mobility-restricted students have great difficulty with such commands.

Prentke Romich markets a keyguard for Apple computers that does everything the IBM keyguard does with Selectrics and also automatically depresses the CONTROL and SHIFT keys as needed. The plastic keyguard costs $110. The price seems inflated until you realize that we are back with the unique diseconomies of scale of "special" equipment, just as with the Autocom.

Vertex Systems has an interesting approach to the keyboard problem. It markets an inexpensive ($45) program called Keyswapper 1.4™, applicable with IBM PC and XT computers. What the program does is enable you to substitute the use of a function key on the keyboard for a string of individual keystrokes. In fact, you can reconfigure the entire keyboard if you wish. Keyswapper 1.4 works with protected and unprotected software suitable for the IBM machines. For more information, contact Vertex Systems (7920 W. 4th St., Los Angeles, CA 90048).

One intriguing application of Keyswapper 1.4 is to change your keyboard to a Dvorak layout. To understand the rationale for doing this, consider the reasons behind the current popularity of QWERTY keyboards (which virtually all typewriters and computers use). The first typewriters (readers old enough to remember the Underwood will know what I'm talking about) were mechanical (manual) rather than electronic. They used a close-packed set of keys, each of which was individually attached to its own striker. To prevent often-used key strikers from interfering with each other on the way to the ribbon, typewriter manufacturers deliberately designed the keyboard so that the most-used keys were widely separated on the keyboard. This brief history lesson explains why the QWERTY keyboard (named after the first six keys on its second row) is so awkward to use. But today's electric typewriters and computers do not face the jamming problem that so worried Milwaukee typewriter inventor Christopher Sholes back in 1873.

According to Virginia Russell, head of Simplified Keyboard Associates of Brandon, Vermont, a typist's fingers travel as many as 16 miles in one day with a QWERTY keyboard. If that is taxing for an able-bodied typist, imagine the problems posed by this archaic setup for students with severely limited mobility.

The Dvorak keyboard, by contrast, requires just one mile's worth of finger travel in the average typist's day, because the most-used keys are placed in the home row of the keyboard. Apple is convinced that the Dvorak layout is worth offering as an option; Digital Equipment Corporation is considering it, according to DEC keyboard design specialist Paul Nelson.

Some keyboard-arrangement programs will combine lengthy strings of commands into one- or two-key functions; others will reconfigure the entire keyboard, even allowing you to custom-design your own. In addition to Vertex Systems, vendors include Advanced Software Interface (2655 Campus Drive, Suite 260, San Mateo, CA 94403), which markets the Keynote™ program; RoseSoft (4710 University Way, NE, Suite 601, Seattle, WA 98105), which offers the ProKey™ program; and Heritage Software (2130 S. Vermont Ave., Los Angeles, CA 90007), which supplies the Smartkey™ program.

Robert Tinker and his associates at Technical Education Research Centers, Inc., are developing an interface to provide access to software designed to run on Atari, Commodore, Apple, and IBM PC computers. Tinker recognizes that students and adults with physical disabilities vary greatly in their capacities. For that reason, his project is concerned primarily with users who cannot key into standard computer keyboards: "Everything special about the user will be contained in the interface itself." The approach, which involves both hardware and software, is expected to be available in mid-1985. For more information, contact Technical Education Research Centers, Inc. (8 Eliot St., Cambridge, MA 02138).

The State of the Art

Two observations may be made about the use of microcomputers in special education today. First, the quality of available software designed to meet the special needs of children, youth, adults, and senior citizens with disabilities is abysmal. Alan Hofmeister, dean of graduate studies and associate vice president for research at Utah State University, who has written extensively on the subject, says: "In general, the quality of presently available educational software is very disappointing." Charles Stallard, associate professor of education at Old Dominion University, adds: "While [computer] experts may understand the technology, they do not understand the needs of teachers and special children. In short, they do not understand the nature of education."

Rather than review the currently available software (which would make dreary reading), I suggest that you contact several organizations that specialize in evaluating commercial and teacher-developed software for use in special-education settings. But keep your expectations modest: you're not likely to find really good special-education software for at least another two or three years.

A good place to start is the National Association of State Directors of Special Education (NASDSE), the organization representing state agency heads. NASDSE is developing training materials for educators, compiling evaluations of hardware and software products, and disseminating information about computer use in special education to professionals in the field. Contact NASDSE (1201 16th St., NW, Washington, DC 20036).

Technical assistance to educators trying to locate software and hardware to meet a particular student's special needs is available from The Network, Inc., an organization that works closely with Educational Products Information Exchange (EPIE) to demonstrate courseware and devices so that local officials (and parents) can make informed decisions. The work of The Network, like that of NASDSE, is supported by a grant from the U.S. Department of Education. Contact The Network, Inc. (290 South Main St., Andover, MA 01810).

Also receiving federal support from the Department of Education is JWK International, a consulting firm. JWK is preparing fact sheets, resource guides, reports, journal articles, and audiovisual materials, together with a data base that supports these products. Parents and educators may tap into this source of information by contacting JWK International, Inc. (7617 Little River Turnpike, Annandale, VA 22003).

LINC Resources, Inc., is facilitating the assessment and distribution of teacher-developed educational software. LINC receives special-education programs, evaluates them for distribution potential, prepares marketing plans for them, and assists their developers to license the programs to commercial and nonprofit distributors and publishers. The importance of this effort is obvious when one considers that the work of Sam Jenkins, of The Upper Room, in developing software for use with retarded and learning-disabled children began as the efforts of an interested parent; it did not start with work by a commercial software publisher. Similar examples could be cited in many other areas of special education. For information about LINC's offerings, contact LINC Resources, Inc. (1875 Morse Rd., Columbus, OH 43229).

Another good source of information is the Council for Exceptional Children (CEC). This remarkable organization has taken a leadership role for many years in bringing special education to its present stage of development. Among many other things available to teachers and parents from CEC are a host of well-written publications and a data base called "ERIC Clearinghouse on Handicapped and Gifted Children." Contact CEC (1920 Association Drive, Reston, VA 22091).

I said I had two observations to make. The second is that the field is clearly ripe for sustained growth. According to Project Tech Mark, conducted by Education Turnkey, Inc., of Falls Church, Virginia, the use of microcomputers will explode in the next three to five years in the special-education field. In a paper entitled, "Market Profile Report: Technology and Special Education," the project staff observed that some 25,000 microcomputers were in use in special education in 1983; by 1986, the number is expected to grow to 150,000. That's a sixfold growth in just three years. The report is available from Education Turnkey (256 N. Washington St., Falls Church, VA 22046-4549).

The U.S. Department of Education National Center for Educational Statistics (NCES), says that 42 percent of the nation's schools had access to one or more microcomputers in 1981. Two years later, NCES reported, their use in elementary schools alone had tripled, from 20 to 60 percent of the surveyed schools. That kind of explosive growth is likely to characterize special education, according to Education Turnkey's Charles Blaschke. He observes that about $10 billion was spent on special education in the 1982–1983 school year. Equally important, he says, is the fact that per-pupil expenditures are 50 percent greater in special education than in regular education.

I mention these data to counter a widespread belief in the commercial software industry: the special-needs market is "too small" to merit serious interest.

Parents have been responsible for much of the growth in the United States and in Europe of special education. Pressure from parents will be needed once again to stimulate the development of appropriate computer-based instruction for students with special needs. P.L. 94-142 provides that American children with disabilities are entitled to a free, appropriate, public education in the least restrictive environment. For children who need or would benefit from personal computers in school, it is possible for parents to suggest that the use of a microcomputer be written into an Individualized Educational Program (IEP) for the child. (The IEP is required by P.L. 94-142, the Education for All Handicapped Children Act; basically, it is a one-year plan that explains how the child will be taught.) In Berkeley, California, for example, Marilyn Head was able to do precisely that for her 16-year-old daughter.

For students in college, university, graduate school, and continuing education programs, section 504 of the Rehabilitation Act of 1973 (P.L. 93-112) provides a means by which needed microcomputers might be made available. Section 504 requires that educational programs benefiting from Federal financial assistance make their offerings "program-accessible," which can mean access to personal computers for individual students. For more information about P.L. 94-142 and section 504, contact Project HEATH (Higher Education and the Handicapped; One Dupont Circle, Washington, DC 20036), and the Project on Science and the Handicapped (American Association for the Advancement of Science, 1776 Massachusetts Ave., NW, Washington, DC 20036).

Growth is particularly needed in software for postsecondary education and continuing education. The software available today in the area of special needs tends to emphasize basic, getting-around-in-stores kinds of skills. There is an urgent need for programs that special-needs individuals can use to acquire more advanced academic and vocational skills—and for hardware accessible to them.

According to a recent survey of the members of the American

Chemistry Society, only one-tenth of one percent of the respondents were visually impaired. David Lunney of East Carolina University attributes the small number primarily to the difficulty blind persons have had in laboratories. He observes, however, that today's chemistry lab courses stress not the visual observation of chemical reactions, but the instrumental measurement of such processes. Why not, then, produce portable laboratory instruments that blind students could use independently to conduct their own experiments? With support from the U.S. Department of Education, that's exactly what Lunney and his colleagues are now trying to do. To find out how well the research is proceeding, contact Lunney at East Carolina University (Greenville, NC 27834).

In Menlo Park, California, Matt Lehmann, who happens to be 75, wrote more than a dozen programs for older students at the Peninsula Volunteers Little House senior center. His students, who range in age from 65 to 86, study languages, politics, and computers themselves. Lehmann found that older people learn better with ordinary instructional techniques than they do with strategies designed for use with children.

That's obvious when you think about it for a few minutes. Sure, the knee-jerk reaction is: "Older people, being conservative and set in their ways, are going to be the last ones to enter the 'computer revolution,' so why study their special needs?" Like many knee-jerk reactions, this one is just plain wrong. Research at the National Institute on Aging, part of the federal National Institutes of Health, has demonstrated that people continue learning well into their eighties and nineties. Lehmann's experiences show that even very old people adapt quite quickly to new technologies.

If anyone in the world knows the intellectual capacities of senior citizens, that person is Mt. Sinai Medical Center's Robert N. Butler, M.D., author of *Why Survive? Being Old in America*, the classic indictment of America's treatment of its mushrooming population of over-65 citizens. A former director of the National Institute on Aging, Butler is unequivocal in his contention that senior citizens can benefit enormously from computer-assisted instruction.

And what are the needs of over-65 persons for accessible hardware and software? Remember that as many as one-third of all senior citizens in the U.S. and probably a similar proportion of over-65 individuals in other countries are disabled. With the remaining two-thirds of the elderly population, hearing and vision may not be severely impaired but they are frequently limited at least to some extent. For example, arthritis and other common age-related conditions may interfere with fine motor control. For all of these reasons, many older people share with younger, disabled individuals what I am calling "special needs."

And—the market is there! The population of people over 65 is growing so fast in the Western world that seniors comprise the single most rapidly expanding group of people in the U.S. and Europe. Given the attractions of The Source, CompuServe, and other data banks, together with the stimulation of learning available through good educational software, and adding into our thinking the fact that millions of older people have large amounts of uncommitted time on their hands, I'm quite willing to predict that the over-65 population will become a major consumer of microcomputer products before ten years have elapsed. I'd make it five years, but personal computers and the software they run are still, despite all the hype, far from "user friendly." I like the analogy made by several Apple executives. Noting that the automobile certainly is complex technology, they sometimes ask visitors to their headquarters if they read the owner's manual when renting a car at the airport. Almost without exception the answer is no.

As the personal computer field becomes more mature, microcomputers, too, will become usable without the need for minute-by-minute reference to bulky "documentation." I don't want to overemphasize the point. While many people who own and rent cars can and do drive them without even looking at owners' manuals, there are problems with such carelessness; it is quite possible to damage a car by using it improperly. Similarly, while I believe strongly that computers need to become more like cars in being interchangeable and in performing similar functions in similar ways, I also recognize that there always will be a need for some documentation. And people drive cars easily because they've grown up with them, seen many others drive them, and feel comfortable with the technologies in them. Perhaps we need to "grow up" with computers in much the same way before they will become as easy for us to use as are cars. Despite these reservations, I do see a trend toward more truly user-friendly computers and I do believe that such machines will attract many more users than do today's products.

People, and especially people with special needs, will use, indeed already are beginning to use, computers not only for education, but for many other tasks as well: doing errands without leaving home, ensuring security in the home, and getting rapid medical assistance in an emergency. These issues form the basis of the next chapter.

CHAPTER 5

INDEPENDENT LIVING

Ever since the word *robot* first appeared (the Czech novelist Karel Capek coined it in 1921), people with special needs have waited longingly for the day when technology would help them live more safely, more securely, more easily, and more conveniently. Physically disabled persons, particularly older people, spend enormous amounts of time, each and every day, handling routine, mundane, maddeningly simple tasks such as turning lights and devices on and off, checking to be sure the home or apartment is secure, handling the shopping, doing the banking, tracking down this piece of information or that. The work takes so long, and consumes so much energy, that precious little time and strength remain to enjoy the day. As the years pass, their worlds become smaller, not larger; concerns about crime, accidents, medical emergencies, and the sheer expenditure of energy required to get through the day make it more and more difficult to live independently. Even so, 90 percent of all Americans over 65 live independently or with family members; only 1.2 million of the 28 million senior citizens live in nursing homes today.

The mushrooming costs of public services for disabled people, older and younger, are forcing difficult choices, particularly in the Scandinavian countries, the United Kingdom, and the U.S. For example, Idaho is now testing a state law that mandates, for the first time, that adult children pay part of their over-65 parents' medical and other care expenses. Idaho's law also says that Medicaid bills for services provided to disabled individuals over the age of 21 are partially the responsibility of their parents. The way was cleared for this law in 1983, when the Reagan Administration issued an interpretation of relevant federal laws, deciding that (if a state had in place a piece of legislation that required families to assume some of the financial obligations of its members) it was lawful for that state to assess adult children of older persons and parents of disabled individuals for some expenses previously assumed by Medicaid. Financial planning expert Jane Bryant Quinn predicts that Idaho's law, if upheld in the courts, will be adopted quickly by the other 49 states.

In Sweden and in the United Kingdom, signs are pointing to a pullback by the state from all-encompassing social programs and a step-up in the state's expectations about family contributions. These trends can only continue and gather momentum because of the ever-larger size of the special-needs population.

Does all of this mean that three-generation households are inevitable? No. Particularly in the U.S., few disabled people want to be an everyday burden on their families. Most, in fact, desire few things more passionately than the ability to live independently, whether that means living with parents or grown children or apart from them: the aim is to direct their own lives without depending on others.

The microcomputer potentially can perform many tasks necessary to permit independent living. With adapted personal computers, many disabled persons can live by themselves and care for themselves much longer than might be possible without these technologies. And in part because the cost of such equipment is decreasing dramatically, there is real hope that the necessary devices will be affordable for individual purchase. For disabled people, many of whom live on restricted incomes, and for adult children (sometimes called "the sandwich generation," because they are caught on one side by the financial and other burdens of their aging parents and on the other side by the pressures of high costs involved in raising children, particularly children with special needs), personal computers may offer a measure of independence and freedom, as well as degree of security once only dreamed about.

Of course, any of these devices will be helpful to people without special needs who want to take advantage of their time-saving, energy-conserving features. In fact, experts predict that by the year 2030, some 80 percent of all households in the U.S. and Europe will handle most of their routine shopping, banking and other financial transactions from the home. As early as 1990, the proportion may be 7 percent or even 10 percent. That's important because, as I have noted earlier, the more people who value products important to disabled individuals, the more likely it is that these devices will be readily available in local stores, easily repaired, and low in cost.

I will start by examining how microcomputers can help special-needs people to handle everyday tasks such as banking, shopping and finding needed information. Then we will turn our attention to the ways in which personal computers can assist in personal security and safety.

Home Banking

In the late 1970s, the Social Security Administration began offering a real service to its tens of millions of American beneficiaries, most of them older or disabled individuals: direct deposit of their monthly checks into their bank checking accounts. Personal computers can take this sensible idea a step further: with a microcomputer, you can handle your bill-paying, check-writing, and other financial transactions from the security of your home. The idea is not as revolutionary as it seems. Banks have offered similar services to business customers for years.

New York's Chemical Bank offers what it calls Pronto. For a monthly fee of $12, you can use your IBM, Apple II or Atari personal computer to do any of the following: balance your checkbook, write checks to about 400 participating merchants if you owe them money, send and receive electronic mail with your bank, and move funds from one account to another. Chemical is demonstrating the Pronto system in participating ComputerLand stores and is offering it to other banks nationwide. To use Pronto, you dial a touch-tone phone to reach a local Tymnet number via your modem. The system then uses special software to help you log on quickly.

Citibank's $10/month Home Base program allows you to use your IBM, Atari, Radio Shack or Commodore computer to pay bills to stores, balance your checkbook, and transfer funds between accounts. As is the case with Chemical's Pronto service, however, you may not make cash deposits or withdrawals. Home Base is expected to be available nationwide late in 1984.

San Francisco's Bank of America provides what it calls Home-Banking for $8 per month. The program accepts input from any personal computer equipped with a modem and a communications package (more about those peripherals in a moment). You can pay bills to some 300 companies and any retail stores to whom you owe money, balance your checkbook, and transfer funds from one account to another, and exchange electronic mail with the bank. HomeBanking uses no special software, an advantage for customers because they need not worry about compatibility between their personal computers and the bank's programs. As with Chemical's Pronto, users call a local Tymnet number to log on with the service. Bank of America has more than 4000 HomeBanking customers in California and plans to expand the service statewide by the summer of 1984.

Other banks planning or already offering home banking include Chase Manhattan, Manufacturers Hanover, and Banc One of Columbus, Ohio. Automatic Data Processing (ADP) in New Jersey, is testing home banking with 20 large and small banks around the country, each of which has between 25 and 200 participating families. Taking part in the ADP project are Chicago's Continental Illinois National Bank and Trust Company, Connecticut's Colonial Bank, Florida's Barnett Banks and New York's Marine Midland Bank.

A large-scale experimental effort is being mounted by Video Financial Services (VFS) that will link Los Angeles' Security Pacific Bank, North Carolina's Wachovia Bank and Florida's Southeast Banking Corporation. These banks are cooperating, through VFS, with the AT&T/Knight-Ridder Viewtron™ experiment, which goes beyond banking to encompass a host of other at-home services. I will talk about Viewtron in the next section of this chapter.

There are a number of advantages and disadvantages to home banking that should be considered. The banks themselves admit that the monthly fees, which range from $5 to $15, are high; your annual investment in fees alone could run as high as $180. Telephone usage fees from your local exchange company and long-distance service are extra. Before making such hefty investments, consider your costs for banking today. If you spend a lot of time getting to and from your bank for routine needs, particularly if you use a cab for these trips, if your mobility is limited, or if your fears for your safety are important concerns, the costs may be worth it.

Two other considerations are privacy and security. There's been a lot of publicity lately about computer freaks breaking into large mainframe computers. With banks, such risks are higher than they are with universities or other institutions because, in Willie Sutton's memorable phrase, "that's where the money is." Most home banking services available today do not "scramble" your communications over the telephone lines with the bank, so the possibility that someone will tap into these messages does exist. If you're an older person, an adult child or another person who knows you well could use the home-banking service to find out about your financial status. Bankers say they take these issues seriously and will implement security procedures before offering the services on a wide scale.

Computers communicate over the telephone by means of what are called "modems" (modulator-demodulators). These come in two kinds: direct-connect, which, as the name implies, you connect directly to your telephone outlet; and acoustic, which have cradles into which you place your telephone handset. Modem costs range from $50 to $450. The higher-cost modems have automatic dialing and other sophisticated features you probably won't need unless you use the equipment a lot. But a modem is not enough. You also need what's called communications software. Such programs allow your computer to send and receive information through the modem. Ask the dealer who sold you the computer for information about compatible programs and modems.

Shopping

A project called Viewtron offers a peek at what's in store for use in years to come. It's an experimental effort offered in Miami, but by the end of 1984 it may be available in other parts of the country at least on a test basis. Viewtron subscribers can handle most of the banking services described above, but they can also do a lot more.

Viewtron is a cooperative venture between AT&T, which provides the terminals (called Sceptre) and Knight-Ridder, which supplies the information (Knight-Ridder is a chain of newspapers and other news media). First, you purchase the $600 Sceptre terminal; you can't use your own home or personal computer with this service, at least not yet. You also pay a $12 monthly fee, plus $1 per hour of use. Viewtron is asking you to make quite an investment. But it's delivering quite a product.

First, let me explain how Viewtron differs from such data base services as The Source and CompuServe. The latter two services are nationwide. Viewtron, by contrast, is local. You receive local news, not just nationwide news. You find out about local stores, local products, local prices. And you can *do* something with the information you see on Viewtron. You can order goods and services; in the Miami test location, you can purchase from more than 100 retailers. E.F. Hutton offers brokerage services, and J.C. Penney provides shopping service for Viewtron customers. Video Financial Services provides banking through Southeast Banking Corp. Not only can you find out what air, rail, bus, and car routes you can take from one place to another, but you can also order tickets for these trips. CompuServe and The Source let you do some of these things, but not with local stores. And Viewtron differs from these services in one other aspect: it gives you, 24 hours a day, full-color depictions of the products, services, and information it describes.

If the project is successful in Florida, Knight-Ridder and AT&T plan to take it nationwide, at least in the locations, such as Detroit, Philadelphia, St. Paul, Charlotte (NC), and San Jose, where Knight-Ridder owns newspapers.

Experiments in the United Kingdom and in France appear to be further along than those in the U.S. In England, British Telecom offers what it calls Prestel to some 20,000 subscribers. Travel information coverage is excellent, offering data on hotels, airlines, restaurants, and other travel-related services. (About one-fourth of Prestel's subscribers are travel agents.) An electronic newspaper is provided, which gives short pieces but not detailed analyses. In France, the federal government distributes, free of charge, Minitel terminals to telephone users throughout the country. All of France is expected to be hooked into the system, which links users to data banks such as telephone number directories, by 1990. One reason for the ambitious plans; the government, which owns the telephone network, thinks it will save a lot of money by providing telephone directories electronically rather than in print. At $175 per terminal, the 400,000 terminals already distributed represent quite an investment by the French government, reflecting its determination to help France commit itself fully to the computer age.

Information

The Source and CompuServe offer one-way communication of information on just about any imaginable topic, drawing on some 1,800 data bases. You can get anything in the *Encyclopaedia Britannica,* any item in the AP or UPI wire services, information from *Books in Print,* data about food and nutrition, and a host of other facts and figures. If these data bases interest you, *Omni Online Database Directory* (Macmillan, 1983) and the quarterly publication *Directory of Online Databases* (Caudra Associates, Santa Monica, CA) may be helpful; both are available in bookstores and in many libraries.

But the most popular services of The Source and CompuServe are their electronic message offerings. If you're an older person with working children, electronic mail would be a convenient way to leave instructions and requests with your peripatetic sons and daughters. No more telephone tag: you type your message on your computer, send it to the service, and check to find your answer a few hours or even a few minutes later.

The Source will be with you for a $100 one-time fee and a $10 monthly minimum usage fee. CompuServe is available for $5 to $23 per hour of use (the higher costs during business hours).

Physically disabled, arthritic, and blind individuals may find the voice-controlled Shadow/VET equipment useful in tapping data bases. Instead of typing as many as 75 or 80 keys in order to tie into the service and locate the information you want, you merely enunciate four or five commands by talking to your computer. For more information, contact Scott Instruments (1111 Willow Drive, Denton, TX 76201). For individuals using an Echo II speech synthesizer from Street Electronics, which permits your computer to talk to you, Bill

Grimm of Computer Aids (4929 South Lafayette St., Fort Wayne, IN 46906) offers software permitting you to hear the information you receive from the data bases. As to the services themselves, you can visit your local computer store for information or write to The Source (P.O. Box 1305, McLean, VA 22101) or CompuServe (5000 Arlington Centre Blvd., Columbus, OH 43220).

Security

Reducing the number of errand trips out of the house will help you feel more secure. Just now coming on the market, though, are some microprocessor-based products that offer rather dazzling services.

Fire is a major concern of older and physically disabled persons; many deaf individuals worry, too, that they will not hear fire alarms. Local phone stores now carry AT&T's Emergency Call System (ECS), consisting of a console ($300) and one or more $30 transmitters activated by your smoke detector. Whether you're home and fail to hear the detector's signal or away from home, the ECS will automatically dial up to two telephone numbers to report the fire, give your address, and request assistance. Before it does all this, however, the unit calls out "Fire" for 30 seconds, during which time you can cancel the transmission (if, for example, you have only burned the toast). AT&T introduced in 1984 an ECS for use in emergency medical signalling ($200): it calls doctors and family members automatically. Coming from Atari, a division of Warner Communications, is an AtariTel home communications system that, company spokesmen claim, will do everything the ECS does plus control appliances and other devices throughout the home.

Basic Telecommunications Corporation offers a remarkable product it calls the AbilityPhone (one word). This unit, which replaces your basic telephone, does all of the following: it serves as a telephone, complete with automatic dialing, directory dialing, automatic redial, and automatic answer; it is a TDD (Telecommunications Device for the Deaf) allowing deaf people to use the telephone by typing rather than talking and listening; it offers environmental control functions, automatically turning on and off up to 16 pieces of equipment (locks, lights, doors, coffeemakers, etc.); it provides the automatic fire-alerting functions offered by AT&T's ECS, calling up to three numbers and announcing (in a synthesized voice) the emergency, your address, and your need for help; it serves as a reminder (saying, in its synthesized voice: "It's time to take your medication"); and, get ready for this feature which I've seen in only one other product: it asks you, at timed intervals (which you set), "Are you OK?" If you fail to respond within five minutes, it automatically dials up to three numbers requesting assistance.

Quite a machine, isn't it? It comes with quite a price, though: $2,735 for the basic equipment, as much as $3,335 fully equipped. A two-year warranty comes with the device. For more information, contact Basic Telecommunications Corporation (4414 East Harmony Rd., Fort Collins, CO 80525).

If you're not quite ready to pay that much for a piece of equipment, consider Phone Care. For just under $500, it will dial up to five numbers automatically if you touch a transmitter worn around your neck or carried in a pocket. Like AbilityPhone, Phone Care will ask if you're all right at predetermined times and automatically issue emergency calls if you fail to respond. For information, contact Newart Electronic Sciences (Twelve Oaks Center, Suite 620, P.O. Box 129, Wayzata, MN 55391).

Or you can use one of the cordless telephones now available to perform a similar service. Some of these are light enough to carry with you in a housecoat or light jacket. Many come, too, with memories you can use to program emergency numbers. If you fall and need help, or feel an attack coming on, just press one button and the phone will do the rest. For details, see your local phone or hardware store.

I've saved Sensaphone for the last, because it's attractively priced ($250) and does things nothing else can do for you. Sensaphone has the capability of monitoring the heat in your apartment or home, the sounds such devices as fire alarms make, electricity use (in case the power goes off), and even such things as a door or window opening. If one of the signals it senses is beyond the level you've determined is acceptable (say, if heat rises above a certain point, one indication of possible fire), Sensaphone automatically calls you or some number you designate, reporting the emergency in a synthesized voice; the system can call as many as four numbers, repeating them in rotation until one answers and acknowledges receiving the message.

With Sensaphone, people can call home to check on temperature, water level in the basement, and a host of other things while being alerted by the machine to any emergency it senses. But older people and physically disabled individuals likely will find it very helpful. Take an example. If your elderly father is susceptible to periodic unconsciousness or periods of inattention to his environment at home, having a Sensaphone call you immediately to report any suspicious sounds or other events would be reassuring. Contact New Horizons (5-31 Fiftieth Ave., Long Island City, NY 11101).

I've mentioned that AbilityPhone will remind you to take your medicine. There's a fascinating, but much less costly, way to handle forgotten dosage requirements. One frequent reason given by families for enrolling an older individual in a nursing home is that the elderly person forgets to take medicine or forgets when he or she last took some pills; the result is either that a condition is not controlled (too few pills are taken) or that an overdose occurs (pills are taken at too-short intervals). Lederle Laboratories offers what it calls a Compliance Aid for Pharmaceuticals (CAP). It's a bottle cap that fits several standard-sized containers. CAP has a digital time readout that displays the day and the time that the cap was last replaced on the container. Each time the patient reopens the container to remove a pill, both date and time reset automatically. By taking the CAP to your pharmacy, you can have your medication placed in a suitably sized container. For more information, contact B.J. Zoltan (Medical Research Division, Lederle Laboratories, Pearl River, NY 10965).

And what about the bugaboo of live-alones, the obscene telephone call? At a local phone store, you can pick up a Fox Fone ($129), which includes a synthesized voice capability. When someone calls you, the ring does not sound until the calling party responds to the artificial voice's request: "Please send my Fox Code." Only if the appropriate three-digit code is given does your phone ring. This means that Fox Fone has to be used by touch-tone callers, because the device does not have speech recognition. If you have a lot of friends who use rotary-dial telephones, you're probably well advised to await introduction of AT&T's Genesis second-generation telephone, which is now in development. There is a Genesis on the market now, but it won't do what we're about to describe. The coming Genesis, observers report, will have speech-recognition capabilities. It will display the caller's phone number on your telephone so you know who is calling. This might discourage obscene callers.

Home Control

Physically disabled people spend many hours each day performing what are for most of us routine tasks. To the extent that these things can be performed automatically, you (or someone close to you) could save an enormous amount of time and energy.

Prentke Romich offers a slew of environmental control units. These ECUs, as they're called, use computer chips to start your coffee in the morning, raise the lights and lower them (gradually or abruptly, at times you choose), answer your telephone, and control just about any other electric or electronic device you designate. Prices vary considerably, depending on what equipment you already have and which functions you desire. You're well advised to ask the company to tell you which individual pieces of equipment you need; one of its consultant vendors may install the system for you. Contact Prentke Romich (8769 Township Rd., 513, Shreve, OH 44676-9421).

If you're adventurous, and if you know something about electronics and about programming in BASIC (the computer language that comes with almost every home and personal computer on the market today), you can do yourself pretty proud with a home control and security system. But be warned: this is not, repeat not, a plug-in-and-go capability.

Unless you're the next Steve Jobs, who founded Apple, or David Packard, cofounder of Hewlett-Packard, you're probably best off purchasing a book to find out what to do and how to do it. SYBEX offers two of the best. Doug Mosher's *Your Color Computer* describes the home-control BASIC program Mosher wrote and the functions of the various devices required. You'll probably spend about $600 or more on the system, which works with the TRS-80 Radio Shack Color Computer™. Apple addicts should read James Coffron's *The Apple Connection* for details on using an Apple computer to control your home. SYBEX also publishes similar books about the VIC 20, IBM PC, and Commodore 64. These books are available in computer stores, bookstores, or direct from the publisher. A third possibility is to contact Jance Associates (P. O. Box 234, East Texas, PA 18046) for information on how to use a VIC 20 or Commodore 64 for home control purposes. Jance, in fact, will sell you a complete system consisting of the home-control package, software you'll need, a written copy of the program, and instructions on how to modify the system to fit your particular needs. The price (exclusive of the computer) is $195: figure on adding another $300 for the home computer (the VIC 20 and Commodore 64 are low in price) and associated peripherals. For Apple II Plus owners, a similar system is available from Compu-Home Systems, Inc. (3333 East Florida Ave., Denver, CO 80210)

What's this all about? Well, author Doug Mosher uses his home-control system to turn lights on and off when he's away to discourage burglars. It automatically controls his outdoor sprinkler and water systems so as to give each plant in his garden exactly the amount of water it needs to grow; his system even checks the amount of water already in the ground around the plants to be sure the soil is not too dry or too wet. It controls the heat in his home, balancing it despite the fact that before he installed his system, some rooms tended to be much cooler and other much hotter than the temperature set on his thermostat. And it starts his coffee in the morning.

Aside from the personal computer, the main elements of Mosher's system are BSR modules and the BASIC program that runs the whole thing. You can pick up a BSR home-control console, a Radio Shack Plug 'n Power (which serves as an interface between the computer and the console), and as many BSR modules (switches that plug into house wiring) as you wish from Radio Shack stores. If you have a Color Computer, the BASIC program you need is in Mosher's book. You'll also need a clock your computer can read, some interface devices, and a lot of patience. Even if you get the books by Mosher and Coffron, or the complete systems from Jance or Compu-Home, you're probably well advised to ask a friend or consultant to help you set up the system.

Another two pieces of advice.

First, you cannot use the system when you're doing something else with your computer. So give serious thought, if you want to computerize your home, to purchasing an inexpensive home computer rather than a sophisticated multipurpose personal computer for this function. Any of the many home computers described in Mosher's *Family Computers Under $200* (SYBEX, 1984) probably would be suitable. Then, for all your other computing needs (word processing, data processing, banking, etc.), use another computer.

Second, if you deviate from your usual routine; going away for a vacation or a business trip, for example; don't forget that your home-control system won't do anything different while you're away than when you're home—unless you tell it to. This is important to remember, because, to take just one example, you don't want coffee starting if no one is home to drink it. Ruined coffee would be the least of your losses. It might help, then, to put an attention-getting sign just inside your front door: "Going Out? Don't forget the Computer Home-Control System!"

Despite all the pitfalls, a personally designed home-control system has a lot going for it. You can set it up to serve *you,* not some hypothetical "average" individual who may be nothing whatsoever like you. You can program your own selections of people to be called if a fire occurs, numbers to be called if a burglary takes place, lights to be turned on or off in what sequence and to what degree of candlepower, what music or other sounds you want to be greeted with in the morning, and what you want a would-be burglar to hear when he or she opens a window or a door. With competent advice, the right equipment, and a good dose of patience, you can design an environment that's fun for you to live in. If you tire of one setup, you can change it.

To get ideas about how to custom-design your own security system, go to your local library and read two interesting articles in *Personal Computing* magazine: "How a Computer Can Control Your Home," by David Gabel, March 1983; and "Loading the Computer for Home Security," by Craig Zarley, October 1983.

Stimulation

Loneliness is a real problem for many older and disabled individuals. I know elderly people who talk to themselves, not because they're senile, but because they want the illusion of human interaction. A personal computer can provide such an illusion. And it can go further: it offers you a gateway to the world, access to thousands of sources of fascinating information you can print out on your computer's printer, connections at reasonable prices to people all over the place for a fraction of direct-connection telephone charges, participation in "party line" chess games and other kinds of conversation about any imaginable topic, and challenge in the form of all kinds of games and software programs.

The personal computer is nonjudgmental; it won't get upset with you if you're in a foul mood. It won't jump at you if you make a mistake (although it most definitely will refuse to function properly until you correct that mistake). It can remember the many bits and pieces of information you need to keep track of but so often forget: people's birthdays, telephone numbers, your old drafts of the "Great American Novel," your nutrition guidelines, and just about anything else.

There's a flip side to all this. Some writers have written dour pieces on the isolation that personal computers are sure to create. By making daily trips to the grocer's or pharmacy unnecessary, these writers say, computers will make older and disabled people even more alone than they are today. I don't believe it. In fact, I think the opposite will occur: you'll be freed from the mundane to interact more often, more enjoyably, and more extensively with people you choose to be friends with, while reducing your exposure to people you'd rather avoid as well as to the dangers of robberies or street accidents. And you'll have more energy for your social contacts precisely because you'll spend less time on routine tasks.

As computers develop further and as prices continue to drop, in a few years you'll find your computer capable of listening to you and responding to what you tell it. It will, in turn, talk to you. Some day, your personal computer will have the capabilities a Sensaphone has today, so the computer will be able to tell how you feel and ask you about it. That's not as fanciful as it might sound; speech recognition is already here. It's a short step to programming a computer with such capabilities so it will recognize the sound of a cough, a sneeze, or a hoarse throat. Speech synthesis, too, already is with us, and at affordable prices, so your computer could ask you when you arrive at your desk in the morning: "Got a cold? I suggest you take two aspirin and see me later." In fact, you may even be able to program your computer to have its own personality: comforting and agreeable, grouchy and touchy, sarcastic and sardonic.

The microcomputer can make you feel more safe and secure, for the very good reason that you will *be* more safe and secure. It can bring far-flung family and friends and needed information closer than ever. It can stimulate your mind, permitting you to continue your education virtually to the day you die. It can free your mind from remembering thousands of details, letting you concentrate on patterns. You will become more creative.

Most important, you'll live independently much longer—and with much more fun.

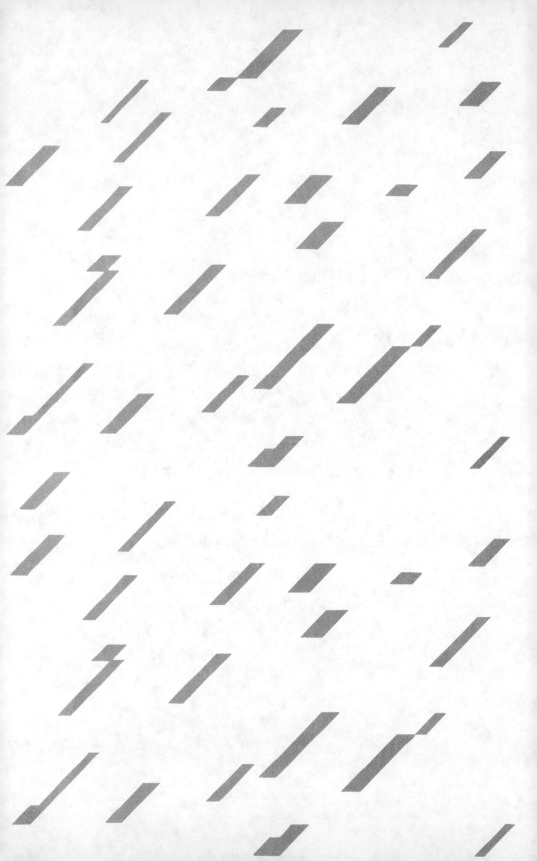

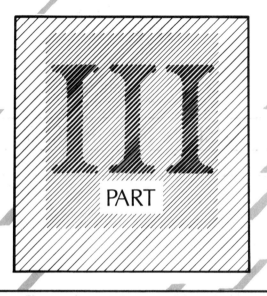

PART

TODAY AND TOMORROW

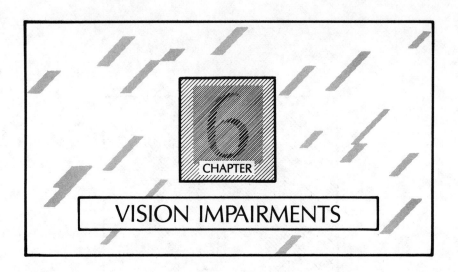

VISION IMPAIRMENTS

When people ask me what microcomputers can do for individuals who are blind, I tell them to get in touch with Judge Leonard Suchanek, a judge with the Board of Contract Appeals in the General Services Administration (GSA) in Washington, D.C. Suchanek is shown in Figure 6.1. A software specialist named Dan Maday set up for Judge Suchanek the single most advanced computer system I've ever seen for persons who are blind.

For starters, Suchanek has a Kurzweil Reading Machine ($29,000, from Kurzweil Computer Products, 185 Albany St., Cambridge, MA 02139). This amazing product reads out loud, in a synthesized voice, virtually any book, memorandum, newspaper, magazine or letter, in any type style or type size imaginable. The user can control the speed of the artificial speech, whether uppercase and lowercase letters should be differentiated vocally, and whether words should be read in toto or spelled out. The price includes training for the user and one year's warranty. The system is not perfect: it pronounces the Judge's name "Such a neck" rather than "Sou hon eck." Such idiosyncrasies are insignificant, though, when you realize that the KRM can not only read anything you want to hear but can also send it into your computer, obviating the need to have someone key in all the information. True, there will be many misspellings; Suchanek is not satisfied with the KRM's 80 percent accuracy rate when used as an automatic entry terminal, preferring to contract out to services that do it with a 98 percent accuracy, but accuracy should improve in the years to come.

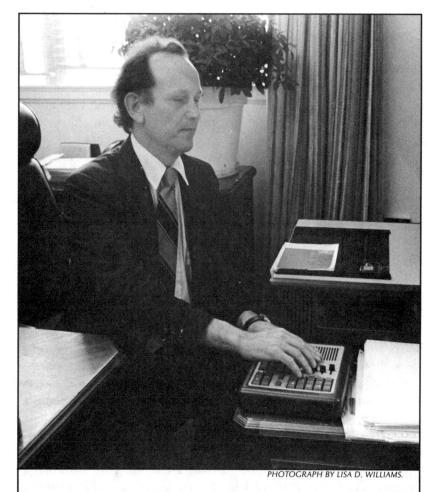

PHOTOGRAPH BY LISA D. WILLIAMS.

Figure 6.1: *Judge Leonard Suchanek operates the Kurzweil Reading Machine in his office. With his right hand he manipulates the controls of the machine; his left hand rests on the book the KRM is reading.*

Judge Suchanek reads Braille. Not all blind people do; most estimates place the proportion reading Braille at under 10 percent of the blind population. Suchanek has an LED-120 Braille printer that takes information from his computer and produces a Braille printout at a staggering 120 characters per second. And this is in top-quality Grade 2 Braille, translated from the English by the system's Duxbury Braille Translator software. The Triformation Systems LED-120, including the Duxbury software, costs about $14,000, but it's falling (the software alone plunged 50 percent in price in 1983).

Next, Maday got for Suchanek and for the GSA a $3,000 Perkins Brailler from Maryland Computer Services. The microcomputer-based machine even looks like the electromechanical original made by the Perkins School for the Blind in Watertown, Massachusetts. It's nice to have around as a portable Brailler. I know blind individuals who arrange with their offices to send information from office word processing machines over the phone lines to the MCS Perkins Brailler so that they can read it themselves rather than have to hire sighted readers to plow through voluminous reports.

Suchanek and Maday weren't done. An Apple work station, complete with modem and various other peripherals, was purchased for $15,000. And, for the office secretarial staff, a DEC minicomputer was added; the Duxbury Braille Translator works with Apple and DEC computers as well as with the LED-120 printer.

Judge Suchanek is the highest-ranking multiple disabled employee in the federal government. He's blind with a partial hearing loss. His work in the Board of Contract Appeals involves an overwhelming reading load. Maday points out that the judge's workload has been reduced by one-third, a considerable savings in the time he needs to review cases and direct the work of the board's lawyers.

The equipment was not purchased for Suchanek's use alone. Maday plans an experimental work station at GSA that will demonstrate microcomputer technology for use by handicapped federal employees in Washington. One person he wants to help: a writer/editor who was left by the effects of Thalidomide with no use of her arms. Maday explained how he was advertising in *Commerce Business Daily* for a special keyboard she could use to write with her feet.

The prices are daunting right now, but they're falling. The LED-120 (illustrated in Figure 6.2) is available from Triformation Systems,

Inc. (3132 S.E. Jay St., Stuart, FL 33494). Maryland Computer Services' Perkins Brailler is available from MCS (2010 Rock Spring Rd., Forest Hill, MD 21050). Apple computers, including a raft of peripherals, may be secured at local computer stores; for the name of the dealer nearest you, contact the company (20525 Mariani Ave., Cupertino, CA 94014).

If your reading requirements run to documents and letters rather than to books and magazine articles, Dest Corporation sells, through local vendors, a $7,000 Dest Workless Station™, which is an electronic document scanner that can read such typefaces as Courier 10 (an IBM Selectric typeface) and seven others. You place a stack of up to 75 pages face up into the machine. Dest's optical character reader "reads" each page, sends the information in digital form ("0" and "1") to your computer, and returns the page, this time face down.

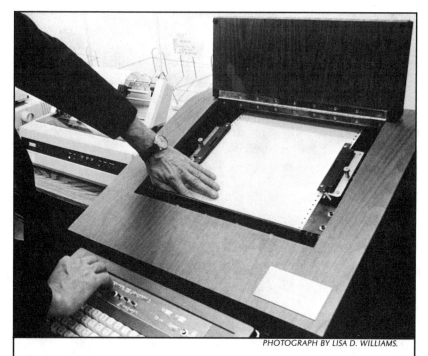

PHOTOGRAPH BY LISA D. WILLIAMS.

Figure 6.2: *Judge Suchanek reads the output of his LED-120 printer, by Triformation Systems, by placing his hand on the paper feed.*

The company claims the machine makes a spelling error once in every 300,000 characters, despite the 25-seconds per page speed. For more information, contact Dest Corporation (2380 Bering Drive, San Jose, CA 95131).

At Vitro Laboratories, a division of Automation Industries, Inc., John Merz, a blind programmer, uses Vitro's special software to do something I thought was impossible: it makes the LED-120 produce three-page-wide graphics that blind people can read. Not everybody wants to emboss missile trajectories and detailed maps like Merz does, but access to graphics is something no other computer system I've seen can provide for blind people. Contact Merz at Vitro Laboratories (1400 Georgia Ave., Silver Spring, MD 20910).

You can get graphics, after a fashion, by using the Optacon device, which reproduces images read by a small camera as tactile impressions you feel with a finger. It's a good machine, popular among blind individuals because it's small, light, and portable. The only problem with the Optacon's graphics capabilities is that you get each small portion of the image, portion by portion, with no overall "picture" of the image. That brings to mind, of course, the proverbial three-blind-men-and-an-elephant joke, but some blind individuals, such as Little Rock, Arkansas, programmer Diana Holzhauser, tell me they can read graphics quite well with the $4,300 Optacon. The device comes with a CRT camera that can be used with "active" computer display terminals. However, the Optacon does not function well with LCD (liquid crystal display) "passive" terminals, such as are now found on computers like the TRS-80 Radio Shack Model 100 portable computer; some experts say that LCD screens are better because they emit no radiation. For information about the Optacon, contact Telesensory Systems, Inc. (3408 Hillview Ave., P.O. Box 10099, Palo Alto, CA 94304).

If you have some residual vision, the extra-large print screens from Visualtek will interest you. Prices range from $2,000 to $4,500 and include the cameras used to read information on another computer if you already have one; if not, Visualtek will provide you with one of its own. Contact Visualtek (1610 26th St., Santa Monica, CA 90404).

Or, if you prefer to listen to information, Maryland Computer Services' Information Through Speech (ITS), at $8,000 (one disk) to $12,000 (Winchester hard disk), is worth looking at. Bill Grimm of

Computer Aids will supply you with a complete hardware-and-software talking system using an Apple IIe and an Echo II speech synthesizer. Grimm's software lets you do word processing, data processing, data base management (including access to The Source and CompuServe data banks), and a lot of other things. Contact Computer Aids, Inc. (4929 South Lafayette St., Fort Wayne, IN 46806).

AVOS offers some interesting software that takes advantage of an Echo GP speech synthesizer to let you do word processing, document formatting, information management, checkbook management, directory filing, and, in your spare time, games. Included in the package are WordStar and CalcStar from MicroPro, programs from Microsoft and AVOS's own voice module and software, and a 64K Z-80 based computer. AVOS lets you use the protected software from MicroPro because it has placed on a board of its own a microprocessor with 512K bytes of buffering. All that technical jargon basically means that the speech synthesizer does not need to use the host computer's operating system, so the problem of interacting with protected software does not arise. The entire package, hardware and software, costs just under $3,000. Contact AVOS, Inc. (1485 Energy Park Drive, St. Paul, MN 55108).

Visually impaired people all over America are getting into computers in a big way. Jeff Weiss and his wife, who live in Little Rock, Arkansas, used Bill Grimm's package of an Apple IIe, Echo II speech synthesizer, and word processing software to write a book on teaching Braille to adults. (American Printing House for the Blind, March 1984.) Larry Scadden, in Washington, DC, uses his computer to manage a private consulting company that specializes in technology for handicapped individuals, and Joe Moore, in New York City, uses his computer to do programming for Manufacturers Hanover Trust.

I also met a young man I'll call Mike. He grew up in Minnesota and moved to Arizona for college. In Tempe, Mike was attending an Arizona State University fraternity party when someone hit him on the head with a heavy wooden board. He spent three months in a coma and, when he awoke, found that he was blind. Mike also has brain damage: his speech is slow and slurred, and he has difficulty remembering some things. Mike is now using an Apple IIe computer and a Model III from Radio Shack to prepare himself to return to work.

For More Information

The American Council of the Blind (1211 Connecticut Ave., NW, Washington, DC 20036) is a consumer organization with chapters in many states. The council is primarily interested in national legislative, judicial, and executive branch decisions affecting blind individuals. It sponsors a number of publications in large print and in Braille; some feature technology applications for blind persons.

The American Foundation for the Blind (15 West 16th St., New York, NY 10011) is a major center of information about blindness. It distributes *Sensory Aids for Employment of Blind and Visually Impaired Persons: A Resource Guide* and other directories of aids.

The Blinded Veterans Association (1735 DeSales St., NW, Washington, DC 20036) is a membership organization primarily consisting of blinded veterans. It publishes newsletters in print and on tape that often discuss the new technologies available for blind persons. Field representatives, themselves blind, are asked to explain to newly blinded individuals, particularly veterans, about new technologies and programs.

The Carroll Center for the Blind (770 Centre St., Newton, MA 02158) conducts research on aids and appliances for blind and visually impaired persons and publishes *Aids and Appliances Review,* a journal designed for American and foreign professionals and consumers concerned with blindness and low vision, which concentrates on U.S. and European resources that perform specific tasks for visually impaired individuals.

Helen Keller International, Inc. (22 West 17th St., New York, NY 10011) works to advance programs for blind individuals worldwide. Its former name is the American Foundation for Overseas Blind, Inc.

The International Association for the Prevention of Blindness (1013 Bishop St., Suite 280, Honolulu, HI 96813) is, despite the name, concerned as much with aids and devices to help blind persons live independently as it is with medical research on preventing the disability.

The Mississippi State University (P.O. Drawer LQ, Mississippi State, MS 39762) conducts research and training on blindness and low vision, seeking ways to help persons live more independently. The program is particularly interested in employment and independent living aids and devices.

The National Association for the Visually Handicapped (305 East 24th St., 17-C, New York, NY 10010) is an information, referral, and service organization primarily interested in persons whose vision impairments are severe, but not total. It publishes newsletters covering topics, including new developments in technology, that affect persons with low vision.

The National Federation of the Blind (1800 Johnson St., Baltimore, MD 21230) is an organization of blind individuals themselves. It publishes *The Braille Monitor,* which looks critically at American programs and organizations serving blind people. The organization helped field-test the Kurzweil Reading Machine in the mid-1970s.

The Pennsylvania College of Optometry (1200 West Godfrey Ave., Philadelphia, PA 19141) conducts research on orientation and mobility for persons with low vision. The project produces a computerized information system of data of interest to researchers, practitioners, and persons who are blind, particularly with respect to mobility aids, hazards, training in the use of aids, and illumination factors in mobility.

The Sensory Aids Foundation (399 Sherman Ave., Suite 4, Palo Alto, CA 94306) publishes a quarterly report documenting advances in the Optacon, a print-to-touch reading system, and other devices. It also distributes, as does the American Foundation for the Blind, *Sensory Aids for Employment of Blind and Visually Impaired Persons: A Resource Guide.*

The Smith-Kettlewell Institute of Visual Sciences (2232 Webster St., San Francisco, CA 94115) is a major rehabilitation engineering center specializing in aids and devices, such as "paperless Braille," for blind individuals.

The Western Pennsylvania School for Blind Children (201 North Bellefield St., Pittsburgh, PA 15213) conducts a project on assessment and treatment with families having visually handicapped children. The work concentrates on counseling and problem-solving strategies as well as referral of appropriate aids and devices.

The World Council for the Welfare of the Blind (58 Avenue Bosquet, 75007 Paris, France) is a major international information source on programs, statistics, and technologies relating to blindness.

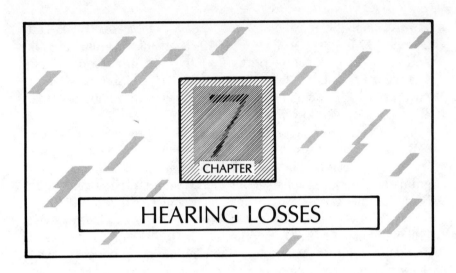

CHAPTER

7

HEARING LOSSES

Steve Rhodes uses his personal computer to study grain shapes in the ocean. The 28-year-old wants to learn the origin of the rocks. "The computer has been a wonderful technological advance for me and my work, because it has helped break down the communication barrier. Working with a computer doesn't require much communication between me and a hearing person." The Columbia, South Carolina, resident is a graduate of Gallaudet College, the liberal arts college for deaf people in Washington, D.C. He lost his hearing when he was 5. His biggest hope? "A company in Atlanta is developing a telephone device which will take what I type and change it to a voice, and then change the other person's voice to printed words." That microcomputer equipment would allow him to use the telephone with people who do not have telecommunications devices for the deaf (TDDs).

Steve is just one of hundreds of thousands of deaf and hearing-impaired people in the U.S. and Europe who use personal computers at work and at home. Of America's 500 school programs serving children and youth with impaired hearing, more than 175 have microcomputers in the classroom. A dozen different companies market

TDDs. One of the latest is Minnesota's Audiobionics, a company founded by the father of a deaf teenager. It does some of the things Steve wants. The device, called a Personal Communicator, includes its own speech synthesizer that translates what a deaf person types into speech, then transmits that spoken message over the telephone wires to, for example, tell parents of a child's whereabouts. The hearing party can respond, using the touchtone buttons on a telephone, "Yes," "No," and the like. The Personal Communicator is small and portable; you can even use it to call your computer at the office. For more information about the $895 device, contact Audiobionics (9913 Valley View Rd., Eden Prairie, MN 55344).

If you want a modem (modulator/demodulator) to use with your TDD so you can call people who own computers, you can get one from Weitbrecht Communications, Inc. The California company was founded by the man generally credited with inventing the original Baudot modem that permits deaf people to use old Teletype machines on the telephone. Robert Weitbrecht is himself deaf. For more information about the Phonetype 1000, contact him (655 Skyway, #230, San Carlos, CA 94070). Intra Computers (101 West 31st St., New York, NY 10001) offers a $200 board to make an Apple computer capable of communicating with a TDD device.

Some of the newer TDDs, like Audiobionics' Personal Communicator, contain the communications capabilities to transmit both ASCII (used by computers) and Baudot (used by TDDs) so you can use your device to talk to anybody who has a TDD or a personal computer. Superphone, from Ultratec, is an example. The light-weight $500 machine, shown in Figure 7.1, has a voice-output option, which adds $400 to the price, making its cost comparable to that of the Personal Communicator. You can also add a printer, an auto-answer feature, and additional memory. For information, contact Ultratec, Inc. (P.O. Box 4062, Madison, WI 53711).

At Rochester Institute of Technology's National Technical Institute for the Deaf (NTID), computers are being used to provide real-time captioning for classroom lectures. When I heard about that, I immediately thought they must have some kind of experimental, continuous-speech-recognition system unavailable anywhere else. After reaching the campus, I learned that the truth was more prosaic. What NTID was doing was to display in the classroom computer-generated printouts of lectures as transcribed by a certified court reporter. As the reporter keyed on a stenotype machine, a computer translated the signals into words, which then appeared on a class-room CRT terminal, one word at a time. The system was experimental. In one test, the words appeared almost simultaneously with the teacher's speech: it is truly a "real-time" system.

I did enjoy, though, listening to the Beatles' song "Yesterday" on a computer at NTID's audio labs. As each word was sung, a small cursor-like indicator bounced over the printed version of the word; through the earphones, I could hear the amplified music as well. Computers are used, too, to provide deaf students with a video image of correct pronunciations against which they can compare similar images of their own speech; this immediate feedback helps deaf students learn to pronounce words and sentence patterns correctly.

In Richmond, Virginia, Ken Macurik has developed a computer-based auditory training unit that works with Apple II+ and IIe

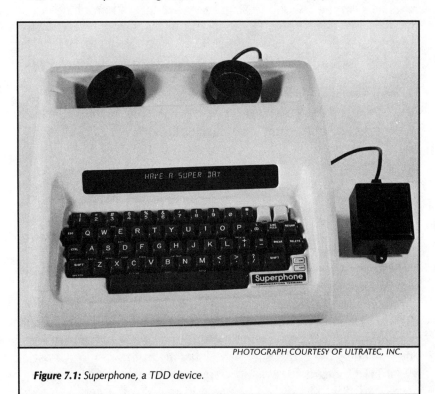

PHOTOGRAPH COURTESY OF ULTRATEC, INC.

Figure 7.1: Superphone, a TDD device.

computers as well as with the TRS-80 Radio Shack Model I. In effect, Macurik's vocalization trainer does the job of a speech therapist. With the Model I, Macurik combines the computer with a Vox Box Radio Shack voice input (speech-recognition) unit and software he wrote. Costs run under $600 for the complete system, including the computer. With the Apple computers, Macurik is using the cassette input port to translate vocalizations. He says that the Apple version offers a higher resolution voice plot, or representation, than does the Model I version. Hearing-impaired persons can compare the visual speech representation they produce against an "ideal" voice plot, gradually making a more exact sound. Contact Macurik (1314 West Main St., Richmond, VA 23284).

The difficulty of mastering the baffling intricacies of the English language is another problem for deaf and hearing-impaired people. I have sometimes compared deafness to being in Tokyo in a sound-proofed glass box. All around you in the bustling streets, people are speaking Japanese, which you do not know but have to learn to survive. Under the circumstances, it is a miracle if you pick up some Japanese words. Mastering the grammar just takes a few years longer! So it is not surprising that many deaf people are somewhat embarrassed about their writing. With so many spelling checkers on the market now, can grammar programs be far behind? A story in *High Technology,* July 1983, shows why there's still quite a way to go. The title tells the story: "Software Tackles Grammar—So Far, Grammar Wins."

The breakthrough for persons with hearing loss (and anyone else who wants help with grammar) may emerge as the AT&T Bell Laboratories UNIX operating system comes into widespread use with 32-bit computers. Dictronics introduced a microcomputer version of one of the Bell Labs Writer's Workbench™ grammar programs late in 1983; it doesn't actually correct your grammar but if you stop typing after hitting the semicolon key, for example, the screen will display the punctuation rules for semicolons.

Wang Electronic Publishing, a division of the Massachusetts company, has a program that will review a letter or chapter you write on your microcomputer, comparing your spelling, punctuation, and use of synonyms and other words against the assembled wisdom of the *Random House Dictionary, Roget's Thesaurus,* the *Chicago Manual of Style,* and *The Elements of Style* by Strunk and White. If you're interested in this electronic English teacher, check it out with Wang Electronic Publishing, Wang Laboratories (1 Industrial Ave., Lowell, MA 08151).

Also worth a look is the Style and Punctuation program from Oasis Systems (3692 Midway Drive, San Diego, CA 92210). Like Dictronics' Grammatik program, it will run on popular personal computers; you don't have to await the 32-bit machines.

But what really gets deaf people excited is speech recognition. It's coming, it's coming. Speech recognition (at least continuous speech, spoken by different people, as opposed to single words by a single speaker, which is available now) may be delayed but it isn't for a lack of effort. All the heavyweights are hard at work on it. AT&T's biggest brains in Murray Hill and Holmdel, IBM's blue-suited geniuses at Yorktown Heights, Control Data Corporation's Minneapolis supercomputer experts, Cray Research's top scientists, and a raft of Japanese specialists are trying to crack the barrier. Edward Fiegenbaum, a top artificial-intelligence expert and coauthor of *The Fifth Generation: Artificial Intelligence and Japan's Computer Challenge to the World,* thinks continuous speech recognition is no more than five to ten years away, given the gigantic commitment of Japanese companies and government to the task. But he hopes American firms can beat Japan to the punch.

Why all the fuss? Several reasons, none of which have anything even remotely to do with helping deaf people. First, continuous speech recognition will let us talk to robots as well as to word-processing machines and data processors, making computers truly "user friendly," if that term has any meaning any more. Second, executives in business are much more likely to take to machines they can talk to than devices they can't understand how to use; the executives sign the checks to multimillion-dollar purchase contracts in business, and that's where the future is for computer companies. General Dynamics and other firms expect that pilots will be able to control aircraft simply by speaking; Unimation thinks "hearing" robots will sell to plants that won't accept "deaf" robots. Perhaps most important in the long run is that speech recognition is a key component of the "fifth-generation" computer, the computer that is supposed to actually learn from its experiences and perhaps even think.

But continuous speech recognition requires enormous amounts

of computer memory. Are we ever going to see it on microcomputers? IBM found, during its initial research on the subject about six years ago, that one hour of time on its largest mainframe was required just to understand one second of speech. Janet Baker, who was with IBM at the time and now heads Dragon Systems, Inc., which specializes in speech recognition, believes that the rapid pace of research since that time has brought continuous speech recognition within sight but that important problems remain. Victor Zue, an expert on speech recognition and one of the few people in the country capable of taking one look at a spectrogram and translating it into the English word that produced it, concedes that researchers have a long way to go before they will solve the riddles of continuous speech recognition.

I'm willing to bet, though, that the complexities of this subject won't defeat one man who moved into the field only three years ago but who may beat them all to the finish line. Up in Waltham, Massachusetts, Raymond Kurzweil is hard at work on a "voice typewriter" with funding support from Xerox and other sources. Kurzweil plans a machine that will take dictation as rapid as 150 words-per-minute and translate it into print. Working with a 10,000-word vocabulary, the machine will accept discrete words after a brief training session. This is the closest anyone has come to date to real continuous speech recognition. While the product is not yet available commercially, indications are that it will be priced for business and educational use, with an initial cost expected to be about $5,000.

Kurzweil is the man who gave us the Kurzweil Reading Machine in 1975. Nine years later, nobody has come close to the KRM's ability to read any typeface or typestyle out loud for blind people. If Kurzweil is successful at his latest venture, he will produce a counterpart for deaf people: a machine that prints what it hears. Write to him at Kurzweil Speech Systems (411 Waverly Oak Rd., Waltham, MA 02154).

For More Information

The Alexander Graham Bell Association for the Deaf (3417 Volta Place, NW, Washington, DC 20007) is an organization primarily comprising parents of deaf and hearing-impaired children and youth, special educators, and speech and language pathologists. AGBAD publishes *The Volta Review,* a journal that reports on technology for special education with hearing impaired persons, developments in hearing aids, and other issues of interest to persons concerned with hearing loss. It also maintains an extensive library of information on devices for persons who are deaf, including TDDs and adapted microcomputers.

The American Association for the Advancement of Science (1776 Massachusetts Ave., NW, Washington, DC 20036) sponsors a Project on the Handicapped in Science and has prepared, for the U.S. Office of Technology Assessment, a recent analysis of communication technologies for deaf persons. AAAS also published *Technology for Independent Living,* a 1982 collection of papers including several on devices for persons with hearing loss.

The American Speech Language and Hearing Association (10801 Rockville Pike, Rockville, MD 20852) is a professional society of speech pathologists and clinicians, language therapists, and audiologists who are particularly interested in special education for children who have speech, learning and language limitations as well as those who have hearing losses. The association publishes a number of professional journals and newsletters and hosts regular professional conventions.

The Clarke School for the Deaf (Round Hill Road, Northampton, MA 01060) conducts research on the use of technology with deaf children, particularly with respect to speech therapy.

Disabled American Veterans (807 Maine Ave., SW, Washington, DC 20024) is an 850,000-member service organization of disabled veterans, which has established, as a key priority, work on behalf of veterans with hearing impairment. DAV publishes a monthly magazine, *DAV,* and hosts national conventions as well as other meetings throughout the year. The organization is in close, continuous touch with the Veterans Administration to advocate for the needs of hearing-impaired and other disabled veterans.

Gallaudet College (Florida Ave. and 7th St., NE, Washington, DC 20002) is the world's only liberal arts college exclusively for deaf people. It maintains an extensive library of information on deafness and sponsors a wide-ranging program of research on technology applicable to meeting the needs of deaf individuals.

The Helen Keller National Center for Deaf-Blind Youths and Adults

(111 Middle Neck Road, Sands Point, NY 11050) is a residential and rehabilitation facility specializing in education, job training, and care for persons who are both deaf and blind. It publishes *NatCent News,* a periodical newsletter, and sponsors research on communication technologies for alerting deaf-blind persons to emergencies and for facilitating interpersonal communication by people who are deaf-blind.

The National Association of the Deaf (814 Thayer Ave., Silver Spring, MD 20910) is one of the oldest consumer organizations formed by disabled individuals themselves. It publishes *The Deaf American,* a magazine, and *The Broadcaster,* a newsletter, both monthly. It also publishes a number of books and audiovisual materials, many of them on sign language. The NAD has chapters in many of America's 50 states.

The National Technical Institute for the Deaf (One Lomb Memorial Drive, Rochester, NY 14623) is located on the campus of the Rochester Institute of Technology. It serves deaf persons interested in a technical education, much as Gallaudet serves those more interested in the liberal arts. NTID also sponsors research on technology, including computers, for instructional use with deaf individuals of college age.

The University of Arkansas (RT-31, 4601 West Markham St., Little Rock, AR 72205) conducts research on postsecondary education and rehabilitation with persons who are deaf or hearing-impaired.

The World Federation of the Deaf (120 via Gregorio VII, 00165 Rome, Italy) is an association of national organizations of persons who are deaf, such as America's NAD. WFD sponsors international conventions every four years.

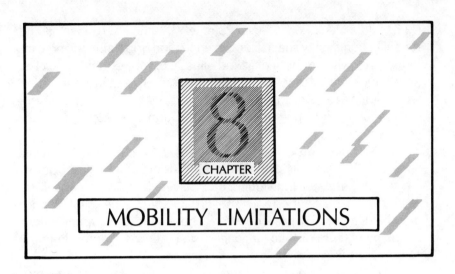

CHAPTER

8

MOBILITY LIMITATIONS

When Gerry Goldberg first went to work for the General Accounting Office (GAO) in Washington, DC twenty-one years ago, his muscular dystrophy was a minor impediment, but today, he needs a powered wheelchair. Even such light exercise as writing or typing can exhaust him. Another disability retirement case, right? Wrong. In 1979, Gerry met Gregg Vanderheiden in Atlanta. As a result of that meeting, Gerry's still at work for GAO.

Vanderheiden showed him how to use an Apple computer and a light pen he wears on his head. If the pen stays on the image of a letter for five seconds, the Apple sends that image through a keyboard emulator, and the appropriate letter appears on the office DEC VT-100 minicomputer. It works—but it's slow. The emulator makes the DEC "think" the letter was typed into its own keyboard.

Gerry prefers working with a large computer, because he need not handle floppy disks or other sensitive materials. The modem he uses to communicate from one computer to another has an auto-dialer feature, so he need not dial telephone numbers. He is constantly "talking" to IBM computers at the National Institutes of

Health, with the DEC computers at the Brookings Institution, and the MICOM systems at other GAO offices in Washington. Gerry reports that he's able to input and manipulate data, run statistical programs, and manipulate text to produce written reports.

Vanderheiden's Trace R&D Center at the University of Wisconsin–Madison maintains a comprehensive data bank on aids and devices such as the light pen Gerry uses. Dr. Vanderheiden also edits the *International Software/Hardware Registry* Trace publishes. And with support from the National Institute of Handicapped Research and Special Education Programs, both of the U.S. Department of Education, he administers several large-scale research and development efforts to improve on existing aids. For more information, contact Vanderheiden (314 Waisman Center, 1500 Highland Ave., Madison, WI 53706).

You can operate an Apple II+ or IIe with just one switch. Adaptive Peripherals markets an Adaptive Firmware Card, which also works with the Franklin Ace computer. With the card in place, users can run off-the-shelf software by manipulating one switch, two switches, or a headwand. Up to 16 different kinds of input may be used, including scanning to locate the desired character or word, Morse Code, direct-selection, "expanded-keyboard" approaches, or assisting features for use with headwands. The card also allows arcade-type games to be played with a game-paddle emulation and a slowdown mode. Installation of the card into an Apple or Franklin computer does not interfere with the use of the computer by someone not taking advantage of the special input features. For more information on the card, which costs about $300, contact Adaptive Peripherals (4529 Bagley Avenue North, Seattle, WA 98103).

A remarkable range of switches can be secured from Prentke Romich (8769 Township Road 513, Shreve, OH 44676-9421).

In Norfolk, Virginia, John Chappell is impressed by the potential of personal computers to help people with severe disabilities. Executive director of Handicaps Unlimited of Virginia, the organization that sponsors Norfolk's Endependence Center, Chappell is an engineer by training and a consumer advocate by preference. He's working with vocal and nonvocal individuals who have severe cerebral palsy to help them learn business skills using TRS-80 Model II and 16 computers. Endependence is one of about a hundred "independent living centers" located in the United States, most of which work with disabled persons in their twenties and thirties.

The major problems, Chappell told me, are those of training people with special needs to use computers and educating employers about what these people can do once they are trained. It's not enough, John stressed, for the equipment to be "out there." Equally important is for persons with special needs to *know* that such things are available; without such knowledge, they too often will think that they are unemployable. Businessmen, too, usually have no idea what can be done with adapted computers—and why it's important to do these things. "We've got to mount a major awareness campaign, coast to coast, to tell people, consumers and employers alike, what's possible with today's technologies," Chappell concluded.

One company that's learned what can be done and is doing its part in spreading the word is Control Data Corporation (CDC). The Minneapolis-based firm, whose chairman Bill Norris is widely regarded as one of the most socially conscious chief executives in the nation, got into the business of adapted computers when several of its key employees became severely disabled. Rather than retire them early, the company looked around to see what it could do to bring them back to work.

The result of years of exploration at CDC is the HOMEWORK™ program. When an employee becomes disabled by an accident or severe illness, a company representative visits with him or her at home or at the hospital. The message: "We're bringing you back." The employee is not permitted to become despondent or to talk himself or herself into believing that return to work is impossible. The next step is assessment of the individual needs presented. Ken Anderson, one of the managers responsible for developing the HOMEWORK program, stresses that each case is different. Once CDC is satisfied it knows what the problems are, two things happen. First, the decision is made about which job the person will perform when returned to work; it may be the previous job, or it may be a different job on the same salary level. Second, the appropriate equipment is assembled and the necessary training begun. Anderson says the usual case takes eight months. More than 50 people, most of them physically disabled, have been returned to work. Of course, PLATO programs, the company's pride and joy, are used to perform the training.

But CDC didn't stop with its own employees. Knowing that many other companies faced similar problems, it set out to market HOME-WORK much as it markets PLATO or its minicomputers. For about $25,000, HOMEWORK staff will perform the entire return-to-work program for another corporation; easier cases cost less, harder ones, more. Corporate executives I've talked to say the program is worth the cost. Not only does the company get a valued employee back on the job, fully trained and ready to go, but such costs as pay for a replacement worker, insurance claim expenses, nonproductive sick pay and other "hidden" expenses are reduced.

Southwestern Bell has taken a different approach. With research support from AT&T Bell Laboratories, California's Telesensory Systems, and other units of what was then the Bell System, Southwestern placed into service new long-distance operator equipment that severely disabled individuals could use. Ann Robson and Tina Heath are two examples of people who wouldn't be employed in their jobs were it not for the investment in new technology. Ann, who's blind, uses Braille and auditory output to keep track of information that other operators monitor by vision. Tina, who is a quadriplegic individual with limited control of her hands and legs, uses a pencil to key information other operators key with their fingers, as shown in Figure 8.1. In both cases, the women were hired, accommodated, and retained in employment because they had something to offer the company: they were good at their jobs. (Note: both women are now with AT&T.)

Trace R&D Center's Gregg Vanderheiden worries, though, that such special equipment might not be so readily available from employers less sensitive to the abilities of special-needs people than are CDC and Southwestern Bell. Vanderheiden concedes that adaptations are possible. A severely disabled person can do just about anything with some computer, particularly if that computer is an Apple or an IBM PC, on which most of the "special-peripherals" work to date has been performed. Physically disabled individuals probably present the greatest challenge, because so many need more than one extra device or add-on to be able to use the computer.

Take the case of someone with severe cerebral palsy who cannot use the standard computer equipment without special adaptations. For this person, an Adaptive Firmware Card, which is compatible with Apple II computers, offers a variety of input options. The card does not interfere with the operation of the computer, so this

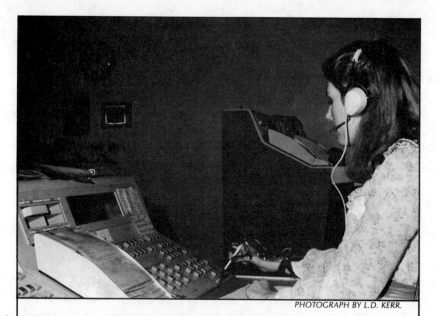

PHOTOGRAPH BY L.D. KERR.

Figure 8.1: *A reasonable accommodation in action. Tina Heath, an operator with AT&T, keys her sophisticated computer-based switching console using a pencil. Quadriplegia limits Tina's fine-motor control, yet she has demonstrated that with a pencil she can match the performance of the company's top operators.*

individual could run standard software on the Apple. Or perhaps an Autocom or Express 3 (both distributed by Prentke Romich) could be used with keyboard emulators that make these special input devices "look" to the Apple like the standard computer keyboard; the Apple can't tell the difference between signals it gets from an Autocom and those it gets from its own keyboard. In some cases, as with Mike Ward, two computers might be used.

The display of sophisticated equipment is impressive. The individual can say: "I can use a computer to do my schoolwork or the work of this job." But, cautions Vanderheiden, what assurance do we have that the school district or employer involved has *these* computers as well? Or that the teacher or office uses *these* software programs? And because of the omnipresent compatibility problems bedeviling the personal computer field, it is fortuitous if the specialized hardware and software are usable in a particular school district or local business. Chances are that one or the other, or quite possibly both, will be incompatible. As Vanderheiden says:

> It is not enough for the handicapped individual to be able to use his own computer and its specially prepared programs. The employer needs workers who can operate the company's computers and its programs. If a disabled person can't do that, then he can't carry out the job. The issue is to equip disabled people to use *standard* hardware and *standard* software that is in place, at the office or at the school or wherever it is that the disabled individual is expected to perform. If we can't do this, then computers will become a new "barrier" for disabled people.

For all of these reasons, Vanderheiden argues, it is not enough to educate people with special needs, on the one hand, and employer and educators on the other, to the capabilities of personal computers in meeting special needs. We must teach, as well, the manufacturers of hardware and software how to make their products accessible to disabled persons. Individuals with mobility limitations are particularly at risk because of their difficulties dealing with the standard keyboards and their need to use the computer for many different purposes, including casual conversation. But blind individuals perhaps are most at risk because of the visual nature of computer terminals. If computer manufacturers can offer these disabled persons ways to use the standard computer, the major problems will be resolved.

Just as buildings had to be made accessible before physically disabled and older people could use them, so too will computers have to become accessible before special-needs persons can become full partners in the computer revolution.

The man I associate most closely with these issues is mathematical statistician Richard Heddinger. In 1972, Dick, then with the U.S. Department of Labor, Bureau of Labor Statistics, filed a lawsuit against the Washington, DC, METRO transportation authority because it was constructing the subway as a system inaccessible to special-needs people. It was a personal issue with Dick, who had polio in the 1954 epidemic. For ten years, he continued the fight. Today, the METRO system is fully accessible.

Dick is now turning to computers. Founder of Janek Computer

Associates, of Bowie, Maryland, Dick is providing technical assistance to corporations that want to purchase computer hardware and software systems. In the pursuit of perfect support services, Janek links its own computer to those purchased by its clients. "We can do the diagnostics after a breakdown, and sometimes fix the problem, without leaving our office," Heddinger says.

What about the accessibility issue? Dick points out that, when he filed his lawsuit, there was a federal law, in fact several of them, specifically requiring that the subway, which was being underwritten by the federal government, be designed to be accessible. It's hard to imagine a more watertight case. Yet several years of heated argument and extended court fights were required before accessibility became a reality.

The key, he believes, is to begin the discussion early in the game. With personal computers still in the Model-T stage, individuals with mobility, hearing, vision, and other special needs should make their desires known to hardware and software manufacturers as quickly as possible. Once investments in equipment and programs become too high, there is massive resistance to going back to "retrofit" so as to meet special needs.

There were many times, Dick says, when it looked as if the METRO subway would not be accessible, even though the law clearly said it had to be. It's something that's worth remembering now that we are facing an accessibility issue of another kind.

For More Information

AbleData (National Rehabilitation Information Center, Catholic University, Eighth and Varnum Streets, NE, Washington, DC 20064) is a computerized information and retrieval service featuring off-line bibliographies and brief descriptions of such aids as signal systems, wheelchairs, and dressing and eating aids for persons with all kind of disabilities. Most of the entries concern persons with different kinds of mobility restrictions.

Accent on Information (Box 700, Bloomington, IL 61701) is another computerized information system, this one operating in response to specific questions posed by users. Coordinated by Cheever Publications, Inc., it maintains an extensive library of information on aids for physically disabled persons and less numerous citations of devices intended for persons with other kinds of impairments. Cheever Publications also issues *Accent on Living,* a consumer publication, and an annual *Buyer's Guide.*

The Baylor College of Medicine (Rehabilitation Medicine Dept., 1200 Moursund Ave., Houston, TX 77030) specializes in research, training, and product development for persons with spinal cord injuries. Lex Frieden, a key figure in independent living, and William Spencer, a leader in technology in medicine, are associated with the program.

Case Western Reserve University (School of Medicine, 2119 Abington Road, Cleveland, OH 44106) works on research to improve the sense of touch in persons with quadriplegia and on other projects in the area of electrical stimulation.

The Cerebral Palsy Research Foundation of Kansas, Inc. (2021 North Old Manor, Wichita, KS 67028) conducts research on worksite modifications that help physically disabled persons to work and investigates robotics, design interfaces with computers, communication devices, and word processors to determine feasibility for use by persons with neurological disorders.

The Electronic Industries Foundation (2001 Eye Street, NW, Washington, DC 20006) works to foster more and better assistive devices for handicapped individuals. It is particularly interested in stimulating private industry to develop and market such aids.

Goodwill Industries of America (9200 Wisconsin Ave., NW, Washington, DC 20814) sponsors sheltered workshops that employ severely disabled individuals and works to enhance their employment in private business.

Human Resources Center (Willets Road, Albertson, NY 11507) conducts research, training, and rehabilitation for severely physically disabled persons and sponsors a sheltered workshop.

International Diabetes Federation (3/6 Alfred Place, London WCIE 7EE, England) offers exchange of information about diabetes and research on ameliorating its effects.

International Federation of Disabled Workers and Civilian Handicapped (Froburgstrasse 4, 4600 Olten, Switzerland) is directed by disabled persons seeking to advance employment for persons with handicaps. It publishes a quarterly, *Bulletin,* and an information sheet, *Nouvelles,* as well as proceedings of its conventions. It is particularly concerned with architectural barriers in the workplace.

International Federation of Multiple Sclerosis Societies (Stubenring 6, A-1010 Vienna, Austria) disseminates information on the condition and research on ameliorating its effects. It publishes (in English, French, and German) *The MS Newsletter.*

Muscular Dystrophy Association of America (810 Seventh Ave., New York, NY 10019) sponsors research on the condition and on ways of helping people with MD live independently.

National Center for a Barrier Free Environment (1015 15th St., NW, Suite 700, Washington, DC 20005) provides information on ways to remove barriers from the built environment. It distributes *Reasonable Accommodation Handbook* and publishes *Report,* a periodical detailing progress toward a barrier-free environment.

National Easter Seals Society (2023 West Ogden Ave., Chicago, IL 60612) coordinates numerous state and local chapters and promotes the use of technologies in employment. It also publishes *Rehabilitation Literature,* a professional journal.

National Multiple Sclerosis Society (205 East 42nd St., New York, NY 10010) advocates on behalf of persons with MS and promotes research into the nature of the condition.

New York University Medical Center (School of Medicine, 500 First Ave., New York, NY 10016) conducts research on neuromuscular diseases including multiple sclerosis.

Tufts University (Dept. of Rehabilitation Medicine, 171 Harrison Ave., Boston, MA 02111) researches nonvocal communication technologies, including visual line-of-sight communication and other corneal-reflection techniques that allow severely disabled persons to use computers and other devices.

University of Pennsylvania (School of Medicine, Dept. of Physical Medicine and Rehabilitation, 3451 Walnut St., Philadelphia, PA 19104) conducts research and training on psychosocial and medical rehabilitation of elderly handicapped individuals, including investigations on early labor-force withdrawal and its effects.

University of Wisconsin (314 Waisman Center, 1500 Highland Ave., Madison, WI 53706) conducts research on access to communication, control, and information processing systems, particularly for nonvocal physically disabled persons. Gregg Vanderheiden is associated with this program.

Yeshiva University/Albert Einstein College of Medicine (1300 Morris

Park, New York, NY 10461) sponsors a Multiple Sclerosis Comprehensive Care Center and a medical rehabilitation research and training center that work on ways to maintain independent functioning in
persons with MS.

CHAPTER 9

LEARNING DISABILITIES

Some of the most dramatic applications of microcomputers occur with children, youth, adults, and older individuals with various kinds of mental limitations.

At the Robert E. Lee High School in San Antonio, Texas, Sandra Jackson, Judy Simmons, and Tony Wedig developed a remedial and diagnostic program for use with a TRS-80 microcomputer. Specifically designed for learning-disabled students, the program helps high school students develop memory, concentration, reading, spelling, and vocabulary skills. They report that because of the program's game-like formats, structured contents, and immediate reinforcement for correct responses, learning-disabled students with attention spans as short as three minutes were able to demonstrate academic growth comparable to that of their able-bodied peers while using the program.

Atari computer games are being used at the Brain Injury Rehabilitation Unit of the Veterans Administration Medical Center in Palo Alto, California. The unit serves veterans with brain conditions due to accidents, strokes, brain tumors, and degenerative diseases. The Atari Hangman game, for example, helps teach spelling by stressing verbal reasoning and logical analysis skills. Brain Game, too, has been found helpful in training patients in memory skills and numerical calculations.

Rosemary Gianutsos and Carol Klitzner, respectively of Adelphi University and Computer Software (Forest Hills, NY), have developed a series of programs designed to run on TRS-80 Model I or III computers. The nine programs help stroke or head-injury patients to recover visual perception and memory skills. Speeded Reading of Word Lists, for example, presents some words left to right, some right to left, and some in the middle of the screen. Reaction Time Measure of Visual Field, another program, displays "runaway numbers" at some point on the computer screen. The patient presses any key to stop the numbers from proliferating. How quickly the user responds, as numbers appear in different positions on the screen, helps therapists diagnose slowed reactions to visual stimuli and design appropriate therapeutic procedures.

I have observed such use in Tel Aviv, where researchers were working with brain-injured veterans and with civilians who had been in severe automobile accidents (both groups are unfortunately large in Israel because of almost continuous warfare in the Middle East and because Israelis tend to be very fast drivers). The idea, I learned, was to force the brain to begin using undamaged cells to conduct the work once performed by the brain cells that no longer functioned properly. Unless information is presented quickly and a response demanded instantly, it is difficult for people to learn to process information in different ways. One of the striking advantages of the microcomputer is that it can offer to the therapists both the required speeded-up images and the immediate measurement of response needed to assess the site of the lesion and to provide appropriate therapy.

In Wisconsin, Sam Jenkins is surprised by the fact that, after nearly two years of work in the application of microcomputers in educating retarded individuals, he still encounters skepticism from parents and teachers that retarded persons can even learn to use a computer, let alone benefit from doing so. Jenkins observes that one of the advantages of personal computers for retarded individuals is the increased attention span that the color animations and speech synthesizers foster. Another is the sense of accomplishment and pride that success in using the computer develops. And learning takes place because feedback is both immediate and nonjudgmental. Often, improved social interaction results when others around the retarded individual praise good work. For more information, contact Jenkins (The Upper Room, 907 6th Avenue East, Menomonie, WI 54751).

In Richardson, Texas, James Muller got so excited about the potential of LOGO, the turtle-based programming language, for learning-disabled and retarded persons that he helped found the Young Peoples' LOGO Association (YPLA), an international group of young people and their parents. YPLA publishes *Turtle News,* as well as a monthly newsletter, *LOGO Newsletter,* aimed at adults, and runs the YPLA Software Exchange, which helps newcomers benefit from the experiences of the "old pros" who still remember the work of Seymour Papert, the MIT mathematician who invented the language.

LOGO is a success with many special-needs individuals because it requires very little language. Manipulation of a "turtle," (triangular-shaped cursor) permits users to draw shapes and conduct "experiments" in geometry. Originally conceived as a way to help children learn to program computers before they were able to read, the language has proven to be effective with people whose mastery of language is restricted. Research at Texas Tech University, for example, demonstrates that LOGO stimulates persistence in children and youth who are "turned off" to many other educational interventions. The children are rewarded immediately for correct actions and gently shown mistakes when these occur. And LOGO offers a unique way to teach abstract concepts to learning-disabled and retarded individuals who have difficulty grasping nonconcrete ideas.

To find out more about this intriguing language, contact the YPLA (1208 Hillsdale Drive, Richardson, TX 75081).

For More Information

The Association for Children and Adults with Learning Disabilities (4156 Library Road, Pittsburgh, PA 15234) is a major organization of state and local chapters consisting largely of parents of children and youth with learning disabilities.

The Autism Services Association (Field School Building, 99 School

St., Weston, MA 02193) conducts research and training in the area of family adjustment and coping strategies for parents and siblings of persons with autism and related disorders.

The Brain Information Service (Center for the Health Sciences, UCLA, Los Angeles, CA 90024) is an excellent data bank of articles and other publications on brain disorders.

The Council for Exceptional Children (1920 Association Drive, Reston, VA 22091) is a major parent and professional organization interested in all aspects of special eduation. CEC publishes *Exceptional Children,* a professional journal that often carries articles on educating children with mental limitations. The organization sponsors national and international conventions, some of which concentrate specifically on the use of microcomputers in special education.

Emory University School of Medicine (1441 Clifton Road, NE, Atlanta, GA 30322) conducts research and assesses technologies in the area of brain injuries.

Epilepsy Foundation of America (1828 L St., NW, Washington, DC 20036) is a national organization of more than one hundred state and local chapters that advocates on behalf of persons with epilepsy, particularly with respect to employment.

The International Association of Workers for Maladjusted Children (66 chausee d'Antin, 75009 Paris, France) sponsors conventions every four years for social workers concerned with enhancing their knowledge about ways to help children who face adjustment problems because of mental, emotional, or other conditions.

The International League of Societies for the Mentally Handicapped (12, rue Forestiere, B-1050 Bruxelles, Belgium) is a major information source and sponsor of international congresses in the area of mental retardation and mental health. It publishes a newsletter in English, French, German, and Spanish.

The National Association for Retarded Citizens (2709 Avenue E East, P.O. Box 6109, Arlington, TX 76011) supports research, training, clinical practice, and education for mentally retarded children, youth, and adults. It is a major international source of information about retardation.

New York University Medical Center (School of Medicine, 550 First Ave., New York, NY 10016) conducts research and training on analysis and treatment of brain trauma, including methods that facilitate the recovery of language use and motor functions.

Northwestern University (Department of Rehabilitation Medicine, 633 Clark St., Evanston, IL 60201) conducts research and training on brain trauma and stroke, particularly on ways to improve educational and vocational performance.

The University of Wisconsin (750 University Ave., Madison, WI 53706) conducts research and training on community integration of mentally retarded individuals, including programs and strategies to help these individuals gain access to postsecondary education and to employment.

The Virginia Department of Rehabilitation Services (Woodrow Wilson Rehabilitation Center, 4901 Fitzhugh Ave., Richmond, VA 11045) works to improve the vocational rehabilitation of learning-disabled adults, particularly with respect to employment.

The World Federation for Mental Health (2255 Wesbrook Crecent, University of British Columbia, Vancouver, BC, V6T 1W5, Canada) publishes *World Mental Health Bulletin,* a quarterly, and many other publications. It serves as a clearinghouse for information and promotes the concept that physical and mental health are intimately related.

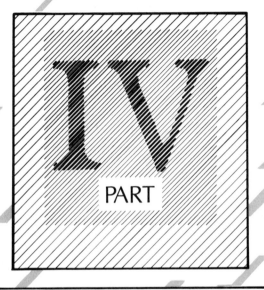

PART IV

WHERE DO WE GO FROM HERE?

CHAPTER 10

RESOURCES AND BUYERS' GUIDE

A good way to get started in the area of microcomputer applications for persons with special needs is to meet some disabled individuals in your area who are using personal computers. Special-needs people using computers are, in my experience at least, more than willing to tell you everything they know—and to show you how to do everything you want to do with a computer.

How do you find these people? One good way is to join a local users' group. For example, several disabled children, adults, and older individuals in the central Arkansas area are members of a local "Apple Addicts" users' group. These organizations usually meet monthly, sometimes in someone's home, more often in a local school or university. Annual fees are modest: $3 for the more rural locations, as much as $15 or $20 in some cities (the New York IBM Personal Computer Users' Group charges $15). Your fees entitle you to attend all meetings and to a newsletter.

Users' groups usually feature a speaker at gatherings, but the emphasis is on what some call "random access" sessions, in which people talk individually about their own interests and the problems they're having with hardware or software. You'll find at least one person in any group who knows how to solve your particular problem, because he or she has run into that problem before. Such "on-the-spot" help can save you a lot of time and aggravation. Many of the larger users' groups have their own subgroups. In New York, for example, the IBM PC users' group has about twenty-five "special interest groups" that meet to talk about topics as diverse as the Pascal programming language and computer graphics, investments and medical applications, word processing and mainframe emulation.

To locate users' groups in your area, contact local computer stores. In fact, when you decide to purchase a computer or some equipment or software to use with a computer, take a few minutes while you're in the store to ask about local users' groups whose members use that hardware or software.

Another good approach is to write to or call your regional or state special-education or vocational-rehabilitation agencies, as well as area programs serving people who are disabled. Area Agencies on Aging (AAAs), too, are an excellent resource. If you are not sure how to find these organizations and agencies, write to one of the national organizations listed in each of the chapters in Part Three. If your child is deaf, for example, a letter to the National Association of the Deaf should bring a quick and helpful response.

Two excellent organizations to contact are the associations representing state directors of special education and vocational rehabilitation.

The National Association of State Directors of Special Education (1201 16th St., NW, Suite 404E, Washington, DC 20036) can direct you to state and local special-education programs. It also sponsors SpecialNet, a computerized information network primarily of interest to special educators, parents, and vocational educators.

The Council of State Administrators of Vocational Rehabilitation (1055 Thomas Jefferson St., NW, Suite 401, Washington, DC 20007) can direct you to state agencies and voluntary associations that can, in turn, help you locate local resources.

State special education and vocational rehabilitation agencies may also provide assistance in the purchase of microcomputers and related aids and software if the student or client qualifies. For information, contact your state agency.

The Veterans Administration (Washington, DC 20420) can direct you to state and area veterans' agencies, hospitals, and organizations. The

VA also can help in purchasing aids for eligible veterans.

If you are interested in postsecondary education, the *Association on Handicapped Student Service Programs in Postsecondary Education* (P.O. Box 21192 Columbus, OH 43221) can direct you to the colleges and universities in your area that offer special support services, including access to computers.

If you're over 55 or know someone who is, the National Council on the Aging (600 Maryland Ave., SW, Washington, DC 20024), the American Association of Retired Persons (1909 K St., NW, Washington, DC 20049), and the National Council of Senior Citizens (925 15th St., NW, Washington, DC 20005) are excellent sources of information about local organizations, agencies, and programs.

If your child is handicapped, you can find out about state and local resources, special programs, and the like by writing to Special Education Programs, U.S. Department of Education (Washington, DC 20201) or to the Council for Exceptional Children (1920 Association Drive, Reston, VA 22091). Ask for the names, addresses, and phone numbers of the resources nearest you.

If you are a disabled individual, contact an organization called COPH-2, sponsored by the Illinois council, Congress of Organizations of the Physically Handicapped. COPH-2 is a geographically dispersed users' group of disabled persons and others interested in special applications with microcomputers (The Committee on Personal Computers and the Handicapped [COPH-2], 2030 Irving Park Rd., Chicago, IL 60618). Request their membership list or ask them to tell you the names, addresses, and phone numbers of persons living near you who are using the kinds of computers you are interested in.

Another way is to go to your local library and leaf through the pages of some of the personal computer magazines. Some, like *Personal Computing* (P.O. Box 2942, Boulder, CO 80322; $18/year), *Family Computing* (P.O. Box 2511, Boulder, CO 80322); and *Popular Computing* (P.O. Box 307, Martinsville, NJ 08836; $15/year) may interest you enough that you will want to become a subscriber. One aspect of these magazines that is often overlooked: their advertising pages often are as informative as are their articles. You can learn about new developments by scanning new-product announcements, then learn more about them by reading critical reviews of the products that interest you.

If you're sophisticated enough to use computer data banks, you may find HEX and EIES/Handicapped helpful.

HEX stands for Handicapped Educational Exchange (11523 Charlton Drive, Silver Spring, MD 20902). It is a clearinghouse for information on the use of technology to help disabled people and to assist in special education. Sources of hardware and software are listed. And, from time to time, conferences take place through HEX by means of which dozens of people from all over the country "talk" to each other via a computerized conference call. As I write, HEX is a free service due in large part to a federal grant, but you must pay your long-distance connection charges.

EIES/Handicapped is a service of the New Jersey Institute of Technology's Computerized Conferencing and Communications Center (323 High St., Newark, NJ 07102). It offers conference calls, electronic mail, report preparation and distribution, and custom-designed communication strategies to let a group come together to discuss a topic electronically. Research on technology for the handicapped is one of the topics on which EIES maintains information. People like Sue Prince, the speech pathologist at the Cerebral Palsy Center in Belleville, New Jersey, pass on to EIES results of the work they do with handicapped children and microcomputers. Costs to use EIES/Handicapped, in addition to your long-distance connection charges, range from $10 to $75 per month plus hourly usage rates.

If you're not sure precisely what you're looking for, a good way to get started is to subscribe to one of several special-interest periodicals. These vary considerably, so I'll describe them in some detail here.

Special Needs Computing (Technical Communications, Inc., 19 Crescent Court, Sterling, VA 22170) is a new monthly publication that covers all aspects of computers and people with special needs. It reviews new products (both specialized and general-market hardware and software); tracks sources of funding, such as special education and rehabilitation agencies that serve disabled individuals and veterans; monitors legislation that affects handicapped individuals; and interviews people who are finding new ways to make computers helpful for people with special needs. This publication is much broader in scope than those that follow; it is also published more frequently. One year's subscription is $48 (U.S.) and $70 (foreign).

The Catalyst (Western Center for Microcomputers in Special Education, 1259 El Camino Real, Suite 275, Menlo Park, CA 94025) is a bimonthly newsletter that carries user-written and other contributed stories about how teachers use computers in special education. Annual subscriptions are $12 (individuals), $20 (agencies, organizations), and $30 (foreign).

Closing the Gap (P.O. Box 68, Henderson, MN 56004) is a tabloid-style newspaper published bimonthly that carries contributed and editor-written pieces on various aspects of using microcomputer technology in special education and rehabilitation with disabled persons. The editor has a special interest in deafness. Annual subscriptions are $15 (U.S.), $22 (Mexico, Canada), and $33 (other foreign).

Communication Outlook (Artificial Language Laboratory, Computer Science Department, Michigan State University, East Lansing, MI 48824) is a quarterly publication reporting on communication aids, assistive devices, and research in the area of work with nonoral, nonverbal, nonvocal, and nonspeech individuals. An annual subsciption is $12.

Bulletin of Science and Technology for the Handicapped (American Association for the Advancement of Science, 1776 Massachusetts Ave., NW, Washington, DC 20036) is a quarterly publication distributed free (for the duration of the federal grant that supports its preparation and distribution) that often includes items dealing with computers.

Other publications that may help you include the *International Software/Hardware Registry,* a loose-leaf binder collection of brief descriptions of computer-related aids and software programs ($15); *Nonvocal Communication Resource Book,* a loose-leaf collection of descriptions of about ninety aids ($20); and *The Rehabilitation Aids Resource Book: Telecommunication, Monitoring, and Environmental Controls,* which includes more than one hundred entries of aids and devices (no price announced), all available from the Trace R&D Center (314 Waisman Center, 1500 Highland Ave., Madison, WI 53706). They are fairly technical, and you may find their entries too brief to be fully understood.

BUYERS' GUIDE TO COMPUTERS AND ADAPTIVE DEVICES

PRODUCT NAME	VENDOR	PRICE (APPROX.)	COMMENTS
Control Units			
AbilityPhone	Basic Telecommunications Corporation 4414 East Harmony Rd. Fort Collins, CO 80525	$2,735–$3,335	Self-contained, multipurpose control and signalling system.
Emergency Call System	AT&T phone centers	$200 for medical emergency signalling, $300 for fire signalling, (plus $30 per transmitter)	Signals to doctors, fire departments, or others designated in advance.
Environmental Control Units	Prentke Romich 8769 Township Rd. Shreve, OH 44676-9421	$600–$1,600	Query vendor regarding personal needs.
Phone Care	Newart Electronic Sciences Twelve Oaks Center, #620 P.O. Box 129 Wayzata, MN 55391	$500	Signals medical emergencies.
Sensaphone	New Horizons 5-31 Fiftieth Ave. Long Island City, NY 11101	$250	Reports heat, sounds, and electricity use via phone. Manufactured by Gulf & Western.

Keyboard-related

Adaptive Firmware Card	Adaptive Peripherals 4529 Bagley Ave. N. Seattle, WA 98103	$300–$350	Emulates keyboard so switches and head-wands may be used; Apple II, II+, IIe compatible.
Autocom	Prentke Romich (address above)	$6,000	Apple compatible; query vendor about other uses.
Keyguard	Prentke Romich (address above)	$110	Fits Apple keyboards.
Keyswapper 1.4	Vertex Systems 7950 W. 4th St. Los Angeles, CA 90048	$50	Lets user "redesign" keyboard or convert to Dvorak layout; IBM PC and XT compatible.
ProKey	RoseSoft 4710 University Way NE Suite 610 Seattle, WA 98105	$130	IBM PC and such "IBM PC compatible" microcomputers as Compaq and Eagle.

BUYERS' GUIDE TO COMPUTERS AND ADAPTIVE DEVICES (CONT.)

Print Readers

PRODUCT NAME	VENDOR	PRICE (APPROX.)	COMMENTS
Dest Workless Station	Dest Corportation 2380 Bering Drive San Jose, CA 95131	$7,000–$8,000	Reads Courier 10 typeface and up to seven others and transfers information to a microcomputer.
Kurzweil Reading Machine	Kurzweil Computer Products 185 Albany St. Cambridge, MA 02139	$29,000	Reads virtually any typeface; synthesized speech.
Optacon	Telesensory Systems 3408 Hillview Ave. P.O. Box 10099 Palo Alto, CA 94304	$2,275	Produces tactile images of print and CRT display.
Voyager	Visualtek 1610 26th St. Santa Monica, CA 90404	$2,000	Enlarges print.

Selected Special Education Software

Title	Source	Price	Description
CHPI Apple Tool Kit	Computers to Help People, Inc. 1221 W. Johnson St. Madison, WI 53715	$15	Interfacing software for Apple II.
Trace Math-Aid	CHPI	$15	Electronic "scratchpad" for Apple II.
Early Counting Fun	The Upper Room 907 6th Ave. East Menomonie, WI 54751	$15	Use with TI 99/4A.
Keyboard Trainer	The Upper Room	$15	Use with TI 99/4A.
Talking Typewriter	The Upper Room	$30	Use with TI 99/4A.

Speech-Recognition Hardware

Title	Source	Price	Description
PC-Mate Voice Recognition Board	Tecmar, Inc. 6225 Cochran Rd. Solon, OH 44139	$995	Use with IBM PC; handles 100 words, expandable to 200 words.

BUYERS' GUIDE TO COMPUTERS AND ADAPTIVE DEVICES (CONT.)

PRODUCT NAME	VENDOR	PRICE (APPROX.)	COMMENTS
Shadow/VET Terminal	Scott Instruments 1111 Willow Springs Dr. Denton, TX 76205	$600	Can recognize 1,000 words in 40-word subsets.
TI Speech Command System	Texas Instruments dealers	$2,200 (plus $600 in additional memory)	Use with TI Professional Computer; recognizes up to 50 words/time.
Voice Input Module	Voice Machines Communications, Inc. 1000 S. Grand Santa Ana, CA 92705	$850–$1025	Use with Apple II, 80-word subsets.
Voice typewriter (generic name)	Kurzweil Speech Systems 411 Waverly Oak Rd. Waltham, MA 02154	To be announced	Query vendor regarding final specifications

Speech-Recognition Software

C2E2	Serota Engineering Consultants 3730 Alta Crest Dr. PO Box 43286 Birmingham, AL 35243	$400	Uses Shadow/VET terminal; Apple II compatible.

Product	Source	Price	Notes
VBLS	Scott Instruments or Swift Publishing 7901 South IH-35 Austin, TX 78744	$100	Authoring system from Swift; uses Shadow/VET. Apple compatible.

Speech-Synthesizer Peripherals

Product	Source	Price	Notes
DECTalk	Digital Equipment Corp. 146 Main St. Maynard, MA 01754	$4,000	Use with most microcomputers.
Echo II	Street Electronics 1140 Mark Ave. Carpinteria, CA 93013	$150	Use with Apple II computers.
Echo GP	Street Electronics	$200	Use with most microcomputers.
Echo PC	Street Electronics	$200	Use with IBM PC.
Ufonic Voice System	Borg Warner Educational Systems 600 West University Drive Arlington Heights, IL 60004	$500	Apple compatible.

BUYERS' GUIDE TO COMPUTERS AND ADAPTIVE DEVICES (CONT.)

PRODUCT NAME	VENDOR	PRICE (APPROX.)	COMMENTS
Type-'N-Talk	Votrax Consumer Products 500 Stephenson Highway Troy, MI 48084	$230	Use with most microcomputers.

Speech-Synthesizer Systems

PRODUCT NAME	VENDOR	PRICE (APPROX.)	COMMENTS
AVOS System	AVOS 1485 Energy Park Drive St. Paul, MN 55108	$3,000	Hardware/software system.
Information Through Speech	Maryland Computer Services 2010 Rock Spring Rd. Forest Hill, MD 21050	$8,000–$12,000	CP/M software compatible talking Hewlett-Packard computer.
Talking Apple	Computer Aids Corporation 4929 S. Lafayette St. Fort Wayne, IN 46806	$1,200–$2,000	Complete system including Apple IIe computer, speech synthesizer, and software.

TDD-related

PRODUCT NAME	VENDOR	PRICE (APPROX.)	COMMENTS
Minicom II	Ultratec P.O. Box 4062 Madison, WI 53711	$150	Inexpensive TDD device that is not computer-compatible.

Programmable I/O board	Intra Computer 101 W. 31st St. New York, NY 10001	$200	Permits Apple computers to communicate with TDDs.
Personal Communicator	Audiobionics 9913 Valley View Rd. Eden Prairie, MN 55344	$900	Computer-compatible TDD that includes speech-synthesizer capabilities.
Superphone	Ultratec	$500	Computer-compatible TDD; speech-synthesizer capabilities are $400 more.

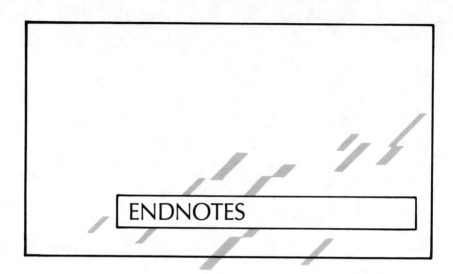

ENDNOTES

I have documented most sources in the text when readability would not be impaired. Following are additional citations by chapter.

Chapter 1

For United Nations data, the demographics are from *The New Internationalist,* "10% of The World's Population is Disabled" (Special Publication, DESI/DEPI, United Nations, New York, NY 10017); for disability by age figures, *Labor Force Status and Other Characteristics of Persons With a Work Disability* (U.S. Bureau of the Census, July 1983, Government Printing Office [GPO], Washington, DC 20402); and for the seniors vs. teens comparison, *Time* (July 11, 1983, pp. 55–56). The reference to governmental costs to keep disabled persons out of the labor force is from *1978 Survey of Disability and Work Data Book* (Social Security Administration, Nov. 1982, GPO, Washington, DC 20402); costs are even higher in most of Europe.

Chapter 2

Demographics are from the U.S. Bureau of the Census publication cited above; from *Handicapping America* (Harper & Row, 1978); and from four publications by the President's Committee on Employment of the Handicapped (all 1984): *Disabled Adults in America, Disabled Women in America, Black Adults with Disabilities,* and *Disabled Adults of Hispanic Origin* (President's Committee on Employment of the Handicapped, 1111 20th St. NW, Washington, DC 20036). See also *America in Transition: An Aging Society* (U.S. Bureau of the Census, Sept. 1983, GPO). Nursing home residence figures are from *Health and Vital Statistics* (National Center for Health Statistics, ser. 14, no. 24, 1981, U.S. Department of Health and Human Services, Washington, DC 20202). Figures on prevalence by type of disability are from *1978 Survey,* op. cit. Joy Schaleben Lewis, a Milwaukee freelance writer, writes about Karen Maliszewski and other youth in "Program Brings Out the Best in Gifted Deaf Teen-Agers" (*New York Times* Education Supplement, Jan. 1983). The work of Dr. Gerald Myers is mentioned in *Personal Computing* (May 1983, pp. 37, 39). Irving Zola writes about his prostheses in "Involving the Consumer in the Rehabilitation Process: Easier Said Than Done," in V. Stern and M. Redden, eds., *Technology for Independent Living* (American Association for the Advancement of Science, 1776 Massachusetts Ave, NW, Washington, DC 20036). On single-task vs. multi-task capabilities, see Gregg Vanderheiden, "Computers Can Play a Dual Role for Disabled Individuals" (*Byte,* Sept. 1982, pp. 136–144). InfoCorp's predictions appear in "Is 'The Real Revolution' in Personal Computers Just Beginning?" (*Business Week,* Oct. 31, 1983, pp. 95–100).

Chapter 3

Lex Frieden discusses his European impressions in "Delivery Systems Abroad" in Stern and Redden, eds. (op. cit., pp. 50–52). Vanderheiden's comments on communication rate appear in "Computers Can Play . . . . " (op. cit.). Herb Brody's piece on computer games appears in *High Technology,* June 1983 (pp. 36–46). For more information about attitudes toward disabled people, see my *Handicapping America* (Harper & Row, 1978). My book, *Reasonable*

Accommodation Handbook, discusses federal legislation and employment-related devices; originally published by AT&T, the book is available from the National Center for a Barrier Free Environment (1015 15th St., NW, Washington, DC 20005). James Raney (American Express), John Reid (Manufacturers Hanover Trust), Edward Corton (Equitable), Richard Drach (DuPont) spoke at the Fifth Annual National Conference on the Industry-Labor Council, Oct. 17–18, 1983, in New York; proceedings from Human Resources Center (Willets Rd., Albertson, NY 11507).

Chapter 4

Nancy Sopp discusses her experiences in a story she sent to *The Catalyst,* a newsletter printed by the Western Center for Microcomputers in Special Education (1259 El Camino Real, Suite 275, Menlo Park, CA 94025). James Muller writes about his son's use of LOGO in "The Birth of the Turtles" (*Closing the Gap,* April/May 1983, p. 5). Margaret Smith is quoted in an AP wire story datelined Harrisburg, PA, June 9, 1983. Andrew L. Ragan cites Sue Prince's beliefs in "The Miracle Worker: How Computers Help Handicapped Students" (*Electronic Learning,* Jan./Feb. 1983, pp. 57–58, 83). Lou Frillman's work at Mill Neck Manor is discussed in *Personal Computing* (Oct. 1983, pp. 253, 256). Eydie Sloane's comments on the Ufonic appear in a mimeographed sheet she sent to fellow "Computer Enthusiasts." Peter Maggs' observations appear in personal communication with me. Sam Jenkins discusses his work in "Research Shows EMR Students Benefit from Computer Use" (*Closing the Gap,* Feb./March 1983, pp. 9, 19). Robert Schadewald offers an excellent overview of speech recognition in "The Speech Gap" (*Technology Illustrated,* June 1983, pp. 55–59). Robb Aley Allen's *Popular Computing* story appears in Oct. 1983 and is entitled: "The Texas Instruments Professional Computer." On the Dvorak keyboard, see "A Keyboard Whose Time Has Come" (*Inc.,* June 1983, pp. 43, 45); the story quotes Virginia Russell. The comments on educational software by Alan Hofmeister appear in *Exceptional Children,* Oct. 1982 (special issue on microcomputers in special education), as do the observations of Charles Stallard. Marilyn Head's success in getting a microcomputer for her daugher in school is mentioned in Mildred Messinger's article, "CP=Computer Proficient" (*The Exceptional*

Parent, Aug. 1983, pp. 57–60). Matt Lehmann's work in Menlo Park is discussed in "The Future is Computer Literacy—At Any Age" (*Personal Computing,* Aug. 1983, pp. 214, 218).

Chapter 5

For an excellent discussion of the safety, security, and health concerns of older disabled persons, see Robert Butler's *Why Survive? Being Old in America* (Harper & Row, 1975). Jane Bryant Quinn writes about the Idaho legistation in "Family Obligations" (*Newsweek,* Aug. 29, 1983, p. 56). *U.S. News & World Report* (Oct. 3, 1983) contains an interview with Stanley Cath that deals with some of the topics raised in this chapter; the title is "If You Have to Care For Your Aging Parents." On home banking, see "Banking Goes Into the Home" (*New York Times,* Dec. 7, 1983, pp. D1, D5); Jane Bryant Quinn, "Banking by Computer" (*Newsweek,* Nov. 21, 1983, p. 85); and *Money* magazine's *Money Guide/Computers* (1983, pp. 56, 58). On shopping, see "A Surprising Eagerness to Sign Up for Videotex" (*Business Week,* April 25, 1983, p. 108); "A One-Stop Shopping Center in Your Home" (*U.S. News & World Report,* May 9, 1983); "Information Services Search for Identity," by Jeff Hecht (*High Technology,* May 1983, pp. 58–65); and "Coming Fast: Services Through the TV Set," by Martin Meyer (*Fortune,* Nov. 14, 1983, pp. 50–56).

Chapter 6

For more information about Judge Suchanek, see John Williams, "Despite Forbidding Handicaps, Justice Triumphs in the Case of Leonard Suchanek" (*People,* Aug. 1983, pp. 50–55). Williams has written many other articles about blind persons using computers (19 Crescent Court, Sterling, VA 22170).

Chapter 7

Kathleen Reid writes about Steve Rhodes in "Independence for Disabled People Through Technology" (*DAV Magazine,* June 1983, p. 12). In addition to Robert Schadewald's "The Speech Gap" (*Technology Illustrated,* June 1983, pp. 55–59), see "Machines That

Think" (*U.S. News & World Report,* Dec. 5, 1983, pp. 59–62); "The Battle of the Supercomputers: Japan's All-Out Challenge to the U.S." (*Business Week,* Oct. 17, 1983, pp. 156–63); "Computers Mastering Speech Recognition," by Andrew Pollack (*New York Times,* Sept. 6, 1983, pp. C1, C7); and "Is 'The Real Revolution' in Personal Computers Just Beginning?" (*Business Week,* Oct. 31, 1983, pp. 95, 99–100). All are excellent sources on various aspects of the work to develop computers capable of recognizing continuous speech.

Chapter 8

An unpublished paper by Gregg Vanderheiden, "Curbcuts and Computers: Providing Access to Computers and Information Systems for Disabled Individuals," discusses some of the ideas presented in this chapter. Persons interested in Control Data Corporation's HOMEWORK program may learn more by writing to the company (8100 34th Ave. South, Box O, Minneapolis, MN 55440). Tina Heath's work is discussed in "Everyone Deserves a Chance" (*Southwestern Bell Scene,* Feb. 1982). For more information on the work for an accessible environment, see my *Handicapping America* and *Rehabilitating America,* both previously cited.

Chapter 9

Texas Tech educators Cleborne Maddux and Dee Johnson discuss "LOGO for the Learning Disabled" (*Closing the Gap,* April-May 1983, pp. 2, 16). Sam Jenkins talks about computers and retarded persons in "Providing CAI for Mentally Retarded" (op. cit., p. 10). Seymour Papert's *Mindstorms* (New York: Basic Books, 1980) is a good introduction to the theory behind the programming language LOGO, written by the authors of the language.

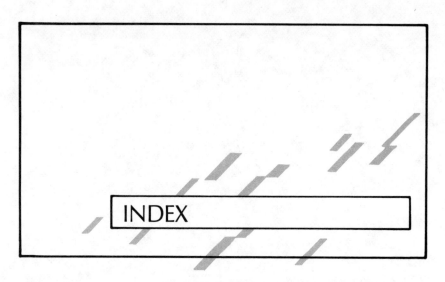

INDEX

Selections from The SYBEX Library

Buyer's Guides

THE BEST OF TI 99/4A™ CARTRIDGES
by Thomas Blackadar
150 pp., illustr., Ref. 0-137
Save yourself time and frustration when buying TI 99/4A software. This buyer's guide gives an overview of the best available programs, with information on how to set up the computer to run them.

FAMILY COMPUTERS UNDER $200
by Doug Mosher
160 pp., illustr., Ref. 0-149
Find out what these inexpensive machines can do for you and your family. "If you're just getting started . . . this is the book to read before you buy."—Richard O'Reilly, Los Angeles newspaper columnist

PORTABLE COMPUTERS
by Sheldon Crop and Doug Mosher
128 pp., illustr., Ref. 0-144
"This book provides a clear and concise introduction to the expanding new world of personal computers."—Mark Powelson, Editor, *San Francisco Focus Magazine*

THE BEST OF VIC-20™ SOFTWARE
by Thomas Blackadar
150 pp., illustr., Ref. 0-139
Save yourself time and frustration with this buyer's guide to VIC-20 software. Find the best game, music, education, and home management programs on the market today.

SELECTING THE RIGHT DATA BASE SOFTWARE
SELECTING THE RIGHT WORD PROCESSING SOFTWARE
SELECTING THE RIGHT SPREADSHEET SOFTWARE
by Kathy McHugh and Veronica Corchado
80 pp., illustr., Ref. 0-174, 0-177, 0-178
This series on selecting the right business software offers the busy professional concise, informative reviews of the best available software packages.

Introduction to Computers

OVERCOMING COMPUTER FEAR
by Jeff Berner
112 pp., illustr., Ref. 0-145
This easy-going introduction to computers helps you separate the facts from the myths.

COMPUTER ABC'S
by Daniel Le Noury and Rodnay Zaks
64 pp., illustr., Ref. 0-167
This beautifully illustrated, colorful book for parents and children takes you alphabetically through the world of computers, explaining each concept in simple language.

PARENTS, KIDS, AND COMPUTERS
by Lynne Alper and Meg Holmberg
208 pp., illustr., Ref. 0-151
This book answers your questions about the educational possibilities of home computers.

THE COLLEGE STUDENT'S COMPUTER HANDBOOK
by Bryan Pfaffenberger
350 pp., illustr., Ref. 0-170
This friendly guide will aid students in selecting a computer system for college study, managing information in a college course, and writing research papers.

COMPUTER CRAZY
by Daniel Le Noury
100 pp., illustr., Ref. 0-173
No matter how you feel about computers, these cartoons will have you laughing about them.

PROTECTING YOUR COMPUTER
by Rodnay Zaks
214pp., 100 illustr., Ref. 0-239
The correct way to handle and care for all elements of a computer system, including what to do when something doesn't work.

YOUR FIRST COMPUTER
by Rodnay Zaks
258 pp., 150 illustr., Ref. 0-045
The most popular introduction to small computers and their peripherals: what they do and how to buy one.

SYBEX PERSONAL COMPUTER DICTIONARY
120 pp., Ref. 0-067
All the definitions and acronyms of micro-computer jargon defined in a handy pocket-sized edition. Includes translations of the most popular terms into ten languages.

FROM CHIPS TO SYSTEMS: AN INTRODUCTION TO MICROPROCESSORS
by Rodnay Zaks
552 pp., 400 illustr., Ref. 0-063
A simple and comprehensive introduction to microprocessors from both a hardware and software standpoint: what they are, how they operate, how to assemble them into a complete system.

Personal Computers

ATARI

YOUR FIRST ATARI® PROGRAM
by Rodnay Zaks
150 pp., illustr., Ref. 0-130
A fully illustrated, easy-to-use introduction to ATARI BASIC programming. Will have the reader programming in a matter of hours.

BASIC EXERCISES FOR THE ATARI®
by J.P. Lamoitier
251 pp., illustr., Ref. 0-101
Teaches ATARI BASIC through actual practice using graduated exercises drawn from everyday applications.

THE EASY GUIDE TO YOUR ATARI® 600XL/800XL
by Thomas Blackadar
175 pp., illustr., Ref. 0-125
This jargon-free companion will help you get started on the right foot with your new 600XL or 800XL ATARI computer.

ATARI® BASIC PROGRAMS IN MINUTES
by Stanley R. Trost
170 pp., illustr., Ref. 0-143
You can use this practical set of programs without any prior knowledge of BASIC! Application examples are taken from a wide variety of fields, including business, home management, and real estate.

Commodore 64/VIC-20

THE COMMODORE 64™/VIC-20™ BASIC HANDBOOK
by Douglas Hergert
144 pp., illustr., Ref. 0-116
A complete listing with descriptions and instructive examples of each of the Commodore 64 BASIC keywords and functions. A handy reference guide, organized like a dictionary.

THE EASY GUIDE TO YOUR COMMODORE 64™
by Joseph Kascmer

160 pp., illustr., Ref. 0-129

A friendly introduction to using the Commodore 64.

THE BEST OF COMMODORE 64™ SOFTWARE
by Thomas Blackadar

150pp., illustr., Ref. 0-194

Save yourself time and frustration with this buyer's guide to Commodore 64 software. Find the best game, music, education, and home management programs on the market today.

YOUR FIRST VIC-20™ PROGRAM
by Rodnay Zaks

150 pp., illustr., Ref. 0-129

A fully illustrated, easy-to-use introduction to VIC-20 BASIC programming. Will have the reader programming in a matter of hours.

THE VIC-20™ CONNECTION
by James W. Coffron

260 pp., 120 illustr., Ref. 0-128

Teaches elementary interfacing and BASIC programming of the VIC-20 for connection to external devices and household appliances.

YOUR FIRST COMMODORE 64™ PROGRAM
by Rodnay Zaks

182 pp., illustr., Ref. 0-172

You can learn to write simple programs without any prior knowledge of mathematics or computers! Guided by colorful illustrations and step-by-step instructions, you'll be constructing programs within an hour or two.

YOUR SECOND COMMODORE 64™ PROGRAM
by Gary Lippman

250 pp., illustr., Ref. 0-152

A sequel to *Your First Commodore 64 Program*, this book follows the same patient, detailed approach and brings you to the next level of programming skill.

COMMODORE 64™ BASIC PROGRAMS IN MINUTES
by Stanley R. Trost

170 pp., illustr., Ref. 0-154

Here is a practical set of programs for business, finance, real estate, data analysis, record keeping and educational applications.

GRAPHICS GUIDE TO THE COMMODORE 64™
by Charles Platt

192 pp., illustr., Ref. 0-138

This easy-to-understand book will appeal to anyone who wants to master the Commodore 64's powerful graphics features.

IBM

THE ABC'S OF THE IBM® PC
by Joan Lasselle and Carol Ramsay

100 pp., illustr., Ref. 0-102

This is the book that will take you through the first crucial steps in learning to use the IBM PC.

THE BEST OF IBM® PC SOFTWARE
by Stanley R. Trost

144 pp., illustr., Ref. 0-104

Separates the wheat from the chaff in the world of IBM PC software. Tells you what to expect from the best available IBM PC programs.

THE IBM® PC-DOS HANDBOOK
by Richard Allen King

144 pp., illustr., Ref. 0-103

Explains the PC disk operating system, giving the user better control over the system. Get the most out of your PC by adapting its capabilities to your specific needs.

BUSINESS GRAPHICS FOR THE IBM® PC
by Nelson Ford

200 pp., illustr., Ref. 0-124

Ready-to-run programs for creating line graphs, complex illustrative multiple bar graphs, picture graphs, and more. An ideal way to use your PC's business capabilities!

THE IBM® PC CONNECTION
by James W. Coffron

200 pp., illustr., Ref. 0-127

Teaches elementary interfacing and BASIC programming of the IBM PC for connection to external devices and household appliances.

BASIC EXERCISES FOR THE IBM® PERSONAL COMPUTER
by J.P. Lamoitier

252 pp., 90 illustr., Ref. 0-088

Teaches IBM BASIC through actual practice, using graduated exercises drawn from everyday applications.

USEFUL BASIC PROGRAMS FOR THE IBM® PC
by Stanley R. Trost

144 pp., Ref. 0-111

This collection of programs takes full advantage of the interactive capabilities of your IBM Personal Computer. Financial calculations, investment analysis, record keeping, and math practice—made easier on your IBM PC.

YOUR FIRST IBM® PC PROGRAM
by Rodnay Zaks

182 pp., illustr., Ref. 0-171

This well-illustrated book makes programming easy for children and adults.

THE COMPLETE GUIDE TO YOUR IBM® PC JUNIOR
by Douglas Hergert

250 pp., illustr., Ref. 0-179

This comprehensive reference guide to IBM's most economical microcomputer offers many practical applications and all the helpful information you'll need to get started with your IBM PC Junior.

DATA FILE PROGRAMMING ON YOUR IBM® PC
by Alan Simpson

275 pp., illustr., Ref. 0-146

This book provides instructions and examples of managing data files in BASIC. Programming designs and developments are extensively discussed.

Apple

THE EASY GUIDE TO YOUR APPLE II®
by Joseph Kascmer

160 pp., illustr., Ref. 0-122

A friendly introduction to using the Apple II, II plus and the new IIe.

BASIC EXERCISES FOR THE APPLE®
by J.P. Lamoitier

250 pp., 90 illustr., Ref. 0-084

Teaches Apple BASIC through actual practice, using graduated exercises drawn from everyday applications.

APPLE II® BASIC HANDBOOK
by Douglas Hergert

144 pp., illustr., Ref. 0-155

A complete listing with descriptions and instructive examples of each of the Apple II BASIC keywords and functions. A handy reference guide, organized like a dictionary.

APPLE II® BASIC PROGRAMS IN MINUTES
by Stanley R. Trost

150 pp., illustr., Ref. 0-121

A collection of ready-to-run programs for financial calculations, investment analysis, record keeping, and many more home and office applications. These programs can be entered on your Apple II plus or IIe in minutes!

YOUR FIRST APPLE II® PROGRAM
by Rodnay Zaks

150 pp., illustr., Ref. 0-136

A fully illustrated, easy-to-use introduction to APPLE BASIC programming. Will have the reader programming in a matter of hours.

THE APPLE® CONNECTION
by James W. Coffron

264 pp., 120 illustr., Ref. 0-085

Teaches elementary interfacing and BASIC programming of the Apple for connection to external devices and household appliances.

TRS-80

YOUR COLOR COMPUTER
by Doug Mosher
350 pp., illustr., Ref. 0-097
Patience and humor guide the reader through purchasing, setting up, programming, and using the Radio Shack TRS-80/TDP Series 100 Color Computer. A complete introduction.

THE FOOLPROOF GUIDE TO SCRIPSIT™ WORD PROCESSING
by Jeff Berner
225 pp., illustr., Ref. 0-098
Everything you need to know about SCRIPSIT—from starting out, to mastering document editing. This user-friendly guide is written in plain English, with a touch of wit.

Timex/Sinclair 1000/ZX81

YOUR TIMEX/SINCLAIR 1000 AND ZX81™
by Douglas Hergert
159 pp., illustr., Ref. 0-099
This book explains the set-up, operation, and capabilities of the Timex/Sinclair 1000 and ZX81. Includes how to interface peripheral devices, and introduces BASIC programming.

THE TIMEX/SINCLAIR 1000™ BASIC HANDBOOK
by Douglas Hergert
170 pp., illustr., Ref. 0-113
A complete alphabetical listing with explanations and examples of each word in the T/S 1000 BASIC vocabulary; will allow you quick, error-free programming of your T/S 1000.

TIMEX/SINCLAIR 1000™ BASIC PROGRAMS IN MINUTES
by Stanley R. Trost
150 pp., illustr., Ref. 0-119
A collection of ready-to-run programs for financial calculations, investment analysis, record keeping, and many more home and office applications. These programs can be entered on your T/S 1000 in minutes!

MORE USES FOR YOUR TIMEX/SINCLAIR 1000™
Astronomy on Your Computer
by Eric Burgess
176 pp., illustr., Ref. 0-112
Ready-to-run programs that turn your TV into a planetarium.

Other Popular Computers

YOUR FIRST TI 99/4A™ PROGRAM
by Rodnay Zaks
182 pp., illustr., Ref. 0-157
Colorfully illustrated, this book concentrates on the essentials of programming in a clear, entertaining fashion.

THE RADIO SHACK® NOTEBOOK COMPUTER
by Orson Kellogg
128 pp., illustr., Ref. 0-150
Whether you already have the Radio Shack Model 100 notebook computer, or are interested in buying one, this book will clearly explain what it can do for you.

THE EASY GUIDE TO YOUR COLECO ADAM™
by Thomas Blackadar
175 pp., illustr., Ref. 0-181
This quick reference guide shows you how to get started on your Coleco Adam with a minimum of technical jargon.

Software and Applications

Operating Systems

THE CP/M® HANDBOOK
by Rodnay Zaks
320 pp., 100 illustr., Ref 0-048
An indispensable reference and guide to CP/M—the most widely-used operating system for small computers.

MASTERING CP/M®
by Alan R. Miller
398 pp., illustr., Ref. 0-068
For advanced CP/M users or systems programmers who want maximum use of the CP/M operating system . . . takes up where our *CP/M Handbook* leaves off.

THE BEST OF CP/M® SOFTWARE
by John D. Halamka
250 pp., illustr., Ref. 0-100
This book reviews tried-and-tested, commercially available software for your CP/M system.

REAL WORLD UNIX™
by John D. Halamka
250 pp., illustr., Ref. 0-093
This book is written for the beginning and intermediate UNIX user in a practical, straightforward manner, with specific instructions given for many special applications.

THE CP/M PLUS™ HANDBOOK
by Alan R. Miller
250 pp., illustr., Ref. 0-158
This guide is easy for the beginner to understand, yet contains valuable information for advanced users of CP/M Plus (Version 3).

Business Software

INTRODUCTION TO WORDSTAR™
by Arthur Naiman
202 pp., 30 illustr., Ref. 0-077
Makes it easy to learn how to use WordStar, a powerful word processing program for personal computers.

PRACTICAL WORDSTAR™ USES
by Julie Anne Arca
200 pp., illustr., Ref. 0-107
Pick your most time-consuming office tasks and this book will show you how to streamline them with WordStar.

MASTERING VISICALC®
by Douglas Hergert
217 pp., 140 illustr., Ref. 0-090
Explains how to use the VisiCalc "electronic spreadsheet" functions and provides examples of each. Makes using this powerful program simple.

DOING BUSINESS WITH VISICALC®
by Stanley R. Trost
260 pp., Ref. 0-086
Presents accounting and management planning applications—from financial statements to master budgets; from pricing models to investment strategies.

DOING BUSINESS WITH SUPERCALC™
by Stanley R. Trost
248 pp., illustr., Ref. 0-095
Presents accounting and management planning applications—from financial statements to master budgets; from pricing models to investment strategies.

VISICALC® FOR SCIENCE AND ENGINEERING
by Stanley R. Trost and Charles Pomernacki
225 pp., illustr., Ref. 0-096
More than 50 programs for solving technical problems in the science and engineering fields. Applications range from math and statistics to electrical and electronic engineering.

DOING BUSINESS WITH 1-2-3™
by Stanley R. Trost
250 pp., illustr., Ref. 0-159
If you are a business professional using the 1-2-3 software package, you will find the spreadsheet and graphics models provided in this book easy to use "as is" in everyday business situations.

THE ABC'S OF 1-2-3™
by Chris Gilbert
225 pp., illustr., Ref. 0-168
For those new to the LOTUS 1-2-3 program, this book offers step-by-step instructions in mastering its spreadsheet, data base, and graphing capabilities.

UNDERSTANDING dBASE II™
by Alan Simpson
220 pp., illustr., Ref. 0-147
Learn programming techniques for mailing label systems, bookkeeping and data base management, as well as ways to interface dBASE II with other software systems.

DOING BUSINESS WITH dBASE II™
by Stanley R. Trost
250 pp., illustr., Ref. 0-160
Learn to use dBASE II for accounts receivable, recording business income and expenses, keeping personal records and mailing lists, and much more.

DOING BUSINESS WITH MULTIPLAN™
by Richard Allen King and Stanley R. Trost
250 pp., illustr., Ref. 0-148
This book will show you how using Multiplan can be nearly as easy as learning to use a pocket calculator. It presents a collection of templates that can be applied "as is" to business situations.

DOING BUSINESS WITH PFS®
by Stanley R. Trost
250 pp., illustr., Ref. 0-161
This practical guide describes specific business and personal applications in detail. Learn to use PFS for accounting, data analysis, mailing lists and more.

INFOPOWER: PRACTICAL INFOSTAR™ USES
by Jule Anne Arca and Charles F. Pirro
275 pp., illustr., Ref. 0-108
This book gives you an overview of InfoStar, including DataStar and ReportStar, WordStar, MailMerge, and SuperSort. Hands on exercises take you step-by-step through real life business applications.

WRITING WITH EASYWRITER II™
by Douglas W. Topham
250 pp., illustr., Ref. 0-141
Friendly style, handy illustrations, and numerous sample exercises make it easy to learn the EasyWriter II word processing system.

Business Applications

INTRODUCTION TO WORD PROCESSING
by Hal Glatzer
205 pp., 140 illustr., Ref. 0-076
Explains in plain language what a word processor can do, how it improves productivity, how to use a word processor and how to buy one wisely.

COMPUTER POWER FOR YOUR LAW OFFICE
by Daniel Remer
225 pp., Ref. 0-109
How to use computers to reach peak productivity in your law office, simply and inexpensively.

OFFICE EFFICIENCY WITH PERSONAL COMPUTERS
by Sheldon Crop
175 pp., illustr., Ref. 0-165
Planning for computerization of your office? This book provides a simplified discussion of the challenges involved for everyone from business owner to clerical worker.

COMPUTER POWER FOR YOUR ACCOUNTING OFFICE
by James Morgan
250 pp., illustr., Ref. 0-164
This book is a convenient source of information about computerizing you accounting office, with an emphasis on hardware and software options.

Languages

C

UNDERSTANDING C
by Bruce Hunter
200 pp., Ref 0-123
Explains how to use the powerful C language for a variety of applications. Some programming experience assumed.

FIFTY C PROGRAMS
by Bruce Hunter
200 pp., illustr., Ref. 0-155
Beginning as well as intermediate C programmers will find this a useful guide to programming techniques and specific applications.

BASIC

YOUR FIRST BASIC PROGRAM
by Rodnay Zaks
150pp. illustr. in color, Ref. 0-129
A "how-to-program" book for the first time computer user, aged 8 to 88.

FIFTY BASIC EXERCISES
by J. P. Lamoitier
232 pp., 90 illustr., Ref. 0-056
Teaches BASIC by actual practice, using graduated exercises drawn from everyday applications. All programs written in Microsoft BASIC.

INSIDE BASIC GAMES
by Richard Mateosian
348 pp., 120 illustr., Ref. 0-055
Teaches interactive BASIC programming through games. Games are written in Microsoft BASIC and can run on the TRS-80, Apple II and PET/CBM.

BASIC FOR BUSINESS
by Douglas Hergert
224 pp., 15 illustr., Ref. 0-080
A logically organized, no-nonsense introduction to BASIC programming for business applications. Includes many fully-explained accounting programs, and shows you how to write them.

EXECUTIVE PLANNING WITH BASIC
by X. T. Bui
196 pp., 19 illustr., Ref. 0-083
An important collection of business management decision models in BASIC, including Inventory Management (EOQ), Critical Path Analysis and PERT, Financial Ratio Analysis, Portfolio Management, and much more.

BASIC PROGRAMS FOR SCIENTISTS AND ENGINEERS
by Alan R. Miller
318 pp., 120 illustr., Ref. 0-073
This book from the "Programs for Scientists and Engineers" series provides a library of problem-solving programs while developing proficiency in BASIC.

CELESTIAL BASIC
by Eric Burgess
300 pp., 65 illustr., Ref. 0-087
A collection of BASIC programs that rapidly complete the chores of typical astronomical computations. It's like having a planetarium in your own home! Displays apparent movement of stars, planets and meteor showers.

Pascal

INTRODUCTION TO PASCAL (Including UCSD Pascal™)
by Rodnay Zaks
420 pp., 130 illustr., Ref. 0-066
A step-by-step introduction for anyone wanting to learn the Pascal language. Describes UCSD and Standard Pascals. No technical background is assumed.

THE PASCAL HANDBOOK
by Jacques Tiberghien
486 pp., 270 illustr., Ref. 0-053
A dictionary of the Pascal language, defining every reserved word, operator, procedure and function found in all major versions of Pascal.

APPLE® PASCAL GAMES
by Douglas Hergert and Joseph T. Kalash
372 pp., 40 illustr., Ref. 0-074
A collection of the most popular computer games in Pascal, challenging the reader not only to play but to investigate how games are implemented on the computer.

INTRODUCTION TO THE UCSD p-SYSTEM™
by Charles W. Grant and Jon Butah
300 pp., 10 illustr., Ref. 0-061
A simple, clear introduction to the UCSD Pascal Operating System; for beginners through experienced programmers.

PASCAL PROGRAMS FOR SCIENTISTS AND ENGINEERS
by Alan R. Miller
374 pp., 120 illustr., Ref. 0-058
A comprehensive collection of frequently used algorithms for scientific and technical applications, programmed in Pascal. Includes such programs as curve-fitting, integrals and statistical techniques.

DOING BUSINESS WITH PASCAL
by Richard Hergert and Douglas Hergert
371 pp., illustr., Ref. 0-091
Practical tips for using Pascal in business programming. Includes design considerations, language extensions, and applications examples.

Assembly Language Programming

PROGRAMMING THE 6502
by Rodnay Zaks
386 pp., 160 illustr., Ref. 0-046
Assembly language programming for the 6502, from basic concepts to advanced data structures.

6502 APPLICATIONS
by Rodnay Zaks
278 pp., 200 illustr., Ref. 0-015
Real-life application techniques: the input/output book for the 6502.

ADVANCED 6502 PROGRAMMING
by Rodnay Zaks
292 pp., 140 illustr., Ref. 0-089
Third in the 6502 series. Teaches more advanced programming techniques, using games as a framework for learning.

PROGRAMMING THE Z80
by Rodnay Zaks
624 pp., 200 illustr., Ref. 0-069
A complete course in programming the Z80 microprocessor and a thorough introduction to assembly language.

Z80 APPLICATIONS
by James W. Coffron
288 pp., illustr., Ref. 0-094
Covers techniques and applications for using peripheral devices with a Z80 based system.

PROGRAMMING THE 6809
by Rodnay Zaks and William Labiak
362 pp., 150 illustr., Ref. 0-078
This book explains how to program the 6809 in assembly language. No prior programming knowledge required.

PROGRAMMING THE Z8000
by Richard Mateosian
298 pp., 124 illustr., Ref. 0-032
How to program the Z8000 16-bit microprocessor. Includes a description of the architecture and function of the Z8000 and its family of support chips.

PROGRAMMING THE 8086/8088
by James W. Coffron
300 pp., illustr., Ref. 0-120
This book explains how to program the 8086 and 8088 in assembly language. No prior programming knowledge required.

Other Languages

FORTRAN PROGRAMS FOR SCIENTISTS AND ENGINEERS
by Alan R. Miller
280 pp., 120 illustr., Ref. 0-082
In the "Programs for Scientists and Engineers" series, this book provides specific scientific and engineering application programs written in FORTRAN.

A MICROPROGRAMMED APL IMPLEMENTATION
by Rodnay Zaks
350 pp., Ref. 0-005
An expert-level text presenting the complete conceptual analysis and design of an APL interpreter, and actual listing of the microcode.

Hardware and Peripherals

MICROPROCESSOR INTERFACING TECHNIQUES
by Rodnay Zaks and Austin Lesea
456 pp., 400 illustr., Ref. 0-029
Complete hardware and software interconnect techniques, including D to A conversion, peripherals, standard buses and troubleshooting.

THE RS-232 SOLUTION
by Joe Campbell
225 pp., illustr., Ref. 0-140
Finally, a book that will show you how to correctly interface your computer to any RS-232-C peripheral.

USING CASSETTE RECORDERS WITH COMPUTERS
by James Richard Cook
175 pp., illustr., Ref. 0-169
Whatever your computer or application, you will find this book helpful in explaining details of cassette care and maintenance.

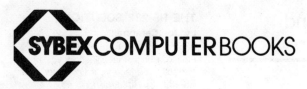

SYBEX COMPUTER BOOKS

are different.
Here is why . . .

At SYBEX, each book is designed with you in mind. Every manuscript is carefully selected and supervised by our editors, who are themselves computer experts. We publish the best authors, whose technical expertise is matched by an ability to write clearly and to communicate effectively. Programs are thoroughly tested for accuracy by our technical staff. Our computerized production department goes to great lengths to make sure that each book is well-designed.

In the pursuit of timeliness, SYBEX has achieved many publishing firsts. SYBEX was among the first to integrate personal computers used by authors and staff into the publishing process. SYBEX was the first to publish books on the CP/M operating system, microprocessor interfacing techniques, word processing, and many more topics.

Expertise in computers and dedication to the highest quality product have made SYBEX a world leader in computer book publishing. Translated into fourteen languages, SYBEX books have helped millions of people around the world to get the most from their computers. We hope we have helped you, too.

For a complete catalog of our publications please contact:

U.S.A.	FRANCE	GERMANY
SYBEX, Inc.	SYBEX	SYBEX-Verlag GmbH
2344 Sixth Street	6–8 Impasse du Curé	Vogelsanger Weg 111
Berkeley,	75018 Paris	4000 Düsseldorf 30
California 94710	France	West Germany
Tel: (800) 227-2346	Tel: 01/203–9595	Tel: (0211) 626411
(415) 848-8233	Telex: 211801	Telex: 8588163
Telex: 336311		